W9-AXN-162

Rail-Trails
Southeast

Rail-Trails: Southeast

1st EDITION September 2006
  7th printing 2013

Maps: Gene Olig and Lohnes+Wright
Map data courtesy of: Environmental Systems Research Institute
Cover design: Lisa Pletka and Barbara Richey
Book design and layout: Lisa Pletka
Book editors: Karen Stewart, Jennifer Kaleba, and David Lauterborn

ISBN 978-0-89997-426-2

Manufactured in the United States of America

Published by: **Wilderness Press**
         c/o Keen Communications
         PO Box 43673
         Birmingham, AL 35243
         (800) 443-7227; FAX (205) 326-1012
         www.wildernesspress.com
Visit our website for a complete listing of our books and for ordering information.
Distributed by Publishers Group West.

Cover photos: Chief Ladiga Trail *(main image)*; McQueens Island Historic Trail
         (upper left); Charlotte Trolley Rail-with-Trail *(lower right)*; Silver
         Comet Trail *(back)*

Title page photo: Cross-Seminole Trail

SAFETY NOTICE: Although Wilderness Press and Rails-to-Trails Conservancy have
made every attempt to ensure that the information in this book is accurate at press
time, they are not responsible for any loss, damage, injury, or inconvenience that may
occur to anyone while using this book. You are responsible for your own safety and
health while in the wilderness. The fact that a trail is described in this book does not
mean that it will be safe for you. Be aware that trail conditions can change from day
to day. Always check local conditions and know your own limitations.

About Rails-to-Trails Conservancy

Headquartered in Washington, D.C., Rails-to-Trails Conservancy (RTC) fosters one great mission: to protect America's irreplaceable rail corridors by transforming them into multiuse trails. Its hope is that these pathways will reconnect Americans with their neighbors, communities, nature, and proud history.

Railways helped build America. Spanning from coast to coast, these ribbons of steel linked people, communities, and enterprises, spurring commerce and forging a single nation that bridges a continent. But in recent decades, many of these routes have fallen into disuse, severing communal ties that helped bind Americans together.

When RTC opened its doors in 1986, the rail-trail movement was in its infancy. While there were some 250 miles of open rail-trails in the United States, most projects focused on single, linear routes in rural areas, created for recreation and conservation. RTC sought broader protection for the unused corridors, incorporating rural, suburban, and urban routes.

Year after year, RTC's efforts to protect and align public funding with trail building created an environment that allowed trail advocates in communities all across the country to initiate trail projects. These ever-growing ranks of trail professionals, volunteers, and RTC supporters have built momentum for the national rail-trails movement. As the number of supporters multiplied, so too did the rail-trails. By the turn of the 21st century, there were some 1,100 rail-trails on the ground, and RTC recorded nearly 84,000 supporters, from business leaders and politicians to environmentalists and healthy-living advocates.

Americans now enjoy more than 13,000 miles of open rail-trails. And as they flock to the trails to commune with neighbors, neighborhoods, and nature, their economic, physical, and environmental wellness continues to flourish.

In 2006, Rails-to-Trails Conservancy celebrated 20 years of creating, protecting, serving, and connecting rail-trails. Boasting more than 100,000 members and supporters, RTC is the nation's leading advocate for trails and greenways.

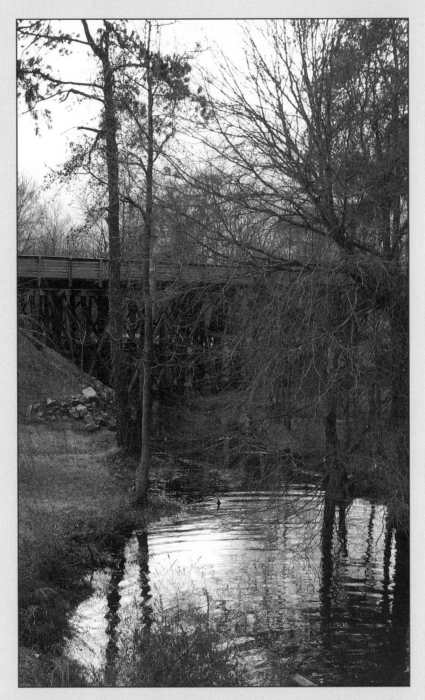

The distinctive cross-bracing of this trestle on the Ten Governors Rail-Trail is a reminder of the trail's railroading past.

Foreword

Dear Reader:

First, for those of you who have already experienced the sheer enjoyment and freedom of riding on a rail-trail, welcome back! You'll find *Rail-Trails: Southeast* to be a useful and fun guide to your favorite trails. It may even help you find some new pathways you didn't already know about.

For you readers who are discovering, for the first time, the adventures you can have on a rail-trail, thank you for joining the rail-trail movement. Since 1986, Rails-to-Trails Conservancy has been the No. 1 supporter and defender of these priceless public corridors, and we are excited to bring you *Rail-Trails: Southeast* so you, too, can enjoy this region's rail-trails.

Built on unused, former railroad corridors, these hiking and biking trails are ideal ways to connect with your community, with nature, and with your friends and family. I've found that rail-trails have a way of bringing people together, and as you'll see from this book, you have opportunities in every state you visit to get on a trail. Whether you're looking for a place to exercise, explore, commute, or play—there is a rail-trail in this book for you.

So I invite you to sit back, relax, pick a trail that piques your interest—and then get out, get active, and have some fun. I'll be out on the trails, too, so be sure to wave as you go by.

Happy Trails,
Keith Laughlin
President, Rails-to-Trails Conservancy

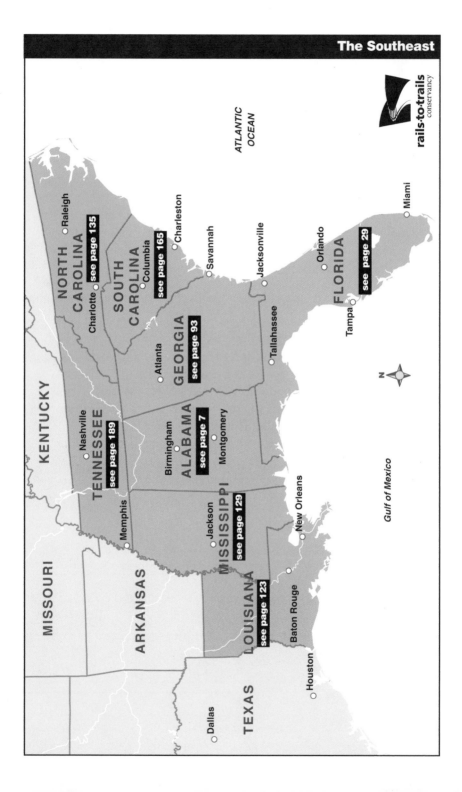

rails·to·trails
conservancy

*ATLANTIC
OCEAN*

NORTH
CAROLINA **see page 135**
○ Raleigh

SOUTH
CAROLINA **see page 165**
Columbia ○

○ Charleston

Charlotte ○

○ Savannah

GEORGIA **see page 93**

Atlanta ○

FLORIDA **see page 29**

Jacksonville ○

Orlando ○

Miami ○

KENTUCKY

TENNESSEE **see page 189**
Nashville ○

ALABAMA **see page 7**
Birmingham ○
Montgomery ○

Tallahassee ○

Tampa ○

Memphis ○

MISSISSIPPI **see page 129**
Jackson ○

New Orleans ○

Gulf of Mexico

LOUISIANA **see page 123**
Baton Rouge ○

MISSOURI

ARKANSAS

TEXAS

Houston ○

Dallas ○

N

Contents

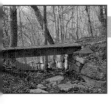

ALABAMA   7

FLORIDA   29

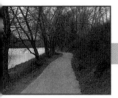

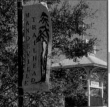

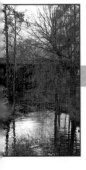

SOUTH CAROLINA · 165

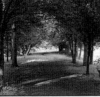

TENNESSEE · 189

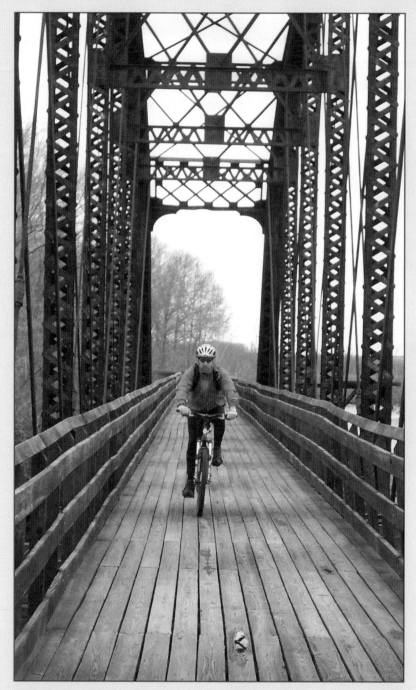

The 550-foot long iron Sycamore Creek Trestle was built in 1903 and is the showpiece of Tennessee's 6.5-mile Cumberland River Bicentennial Trail.

INTRODUCTION

Of the nearly 1,400 rail-trails across the United States, 114 thread through the Southeast states of Alabama, Florida, Georgia, Louisiana, Mississippi, North Carolina, South Carolina, and Tennessee. These routes relate a two-part story: The first speaks to the early years of railroading, while the second showcases efforts by Rails-to-Trails Conservancy, community groups, and their supporters to resurrect these unused railroad corridors as public-use trails.

Rail-Trails: Southeast highlights 55 of the region's diverse trails, each serving as a window on the communities the railroad once served. Some trails delve into the particular history of an area, such as North Carolina's mile-long Gold Hill Rail-Trail. Others offer an escape from city life, such as Georgia's Silver Comet Trail, which runs 50 miles from Atlanta's suburbs to the Alabama state line.

Florida leads the pack with 35 rail-trails that crisscross more than 300 miles. Among them is the 34-mile Fred Marquis Pinellas Trail, one of the country's most popular rail-trails, which welcomes more than 1 million annual visitors. The future of the Sunshine State's trail movement is bright, with 40 pending rail-trail projects that would add more than 500 miles to the state's existing network.

Though Mississippi claims only four rail-trails and Louisiana just one, each state has put considerable effort into making its trails memorable. Mississippi's 41-mile Longleaf Trace leads from the University of Southern Mississippi campus in Hattiesburg through neighborhoods into fragrant piney woods and small-town countryside. Having weathered Hurricane Katrina, southern Louisiana's 27.5-mile Tammany Trace takes a spin through the bayous.

Alabama's offerings range from the varied 33-mile Chief Ladiga Trail, which crosses both Talladega National Forest and the Jacksonville State University campus, to the mile-long Vulcan Trail, which summits 1,025-foot Red Mountain and overlooks Birmingham's storied Civil Rights District.

Among the country's oldest rail-trails is the 0.8-mile Cathedral Aisle Trail, in Aiken, South Carolina, which was converted in September 1939. The corridor it occupies was once the world's longest rail line. Another rail-trail rife with history is the Cumberland River Bicentennial Trail, just outside Nashville, Tennessee. Stroll it for languid river views and look for initials etched into the limestone bluffs back in the 1930s when the railroad was in operation.

1

No matter which route in *Rail-Trails: Southeast* you decide to ply, you'll be touching on the heart of the community that helped build it and the history that first brought the rails to the region.

What is a Rail-Trail?

Rail-trails are multiuse public paths built along former railroad corridors. Most often flat or following a gentle grade, they are suited to walking, running, cycling, mountain biking, inline skating, cross-country skiing, horseback riding, and wheelchair use. Since the 1960s, Americans have created more than 13,000 miles of rail-trails throughout the country.

These extremely popular recreation and transportation corridors traverse urban, suburban, and rural landscapes. Many preserve historic landmarks, while others serve as wildlife conservation corridors, linking isolated parks and establishing greenways in developed areas. Rail-trails also stimulate local economies by boosting tourism and promoting trailside businesses.

What is a Rail-with-Trail?

A rail-with-trail is a public path that parallels a still-active rail line. Some run adjacent to high-speed, scheduled trains, often linking public transportation stations, while others follow tourist routes and slow-moving excursion trains. Many share an easement, separated from the rails by extensive fencing. There are more than 115 rails-with-trails in the U.S.

HOW TO USE THIS BOOK

*R*ail-Trails: Southeast provides the information you'll need to plan a rewarding rail-trail trek. With words to inspire you and maps to chart your path, it makes choosing the best route a breeze. Following are some of the highlights.

Maps

You'll find three levels of maps in this book: an **overall regional map**, **state locator maps**, and **detailed trail maps**.

The Southeast region includes Alabama, Florida, Georgia, Louisiana, Mississippi, North Carolina, South Carolina, and Tennessee. Each chapter details a particular state's network of trails, marked on locator maps in the chapter introduction. Use these maps to find the trails nearest you, or select several neighboring trails and plan a weekend hiking or biking excursion. Once you find a trail on a state locator map, simply flip to the corresponding page number for a full description. Accompanying trail maps mark each route's access roads, trailheads, parking areas, restrooms, and other defining features.

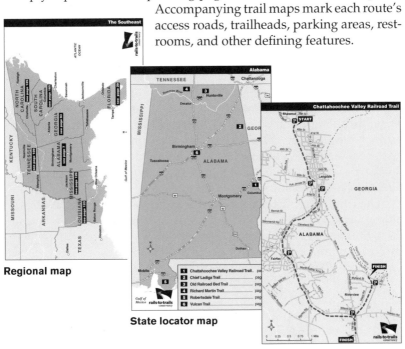

Regional map

State locator map

Trail map

Trail Descriptions

Trails are listed in alphabetical order within each chapter. Each description leads off with a set of summary information, including trail endpoints and mileage, a roughness index, the trail surface, and possible uses.

The map and summary information list the trail endpoints (either a city, street, or more specific location), with suggested points from which to start and finish. Additional access points are marked on the maps and mentioned in the trail descriptions. The maps and descriptions also highlight available amenities, including parking and restrooms, as well as such area attractions as shops, services, museums, parks, and stadiums. Trail length is listed in miles.

Each trail bears a roughness index rating from 1 to 3. A rating of 1 indicates a smooth, level surface that is accessible to users of all ages and abilities. A 2 rating means the surface may be loose and/or uneven and could pose a problem for road bikes and wheelchairs. A 3 rating suggests a rough surface that is only recommended for mountain bikers and hikers. Surfaces can range from asphalt or concrete to ballast, cinder, crushed stone, gravel, grass, dirt, and/or sand. Where relevant, trail descriptions address alternating surface conditions.

All rail-trails are open to pedestrians, and most allow bicycles, except where noted in the trail summary or description. The summary also indicates wheelchair access. Other possible uses include inline skating, cycling, mountain biking, hiking, horseback riding, fishing, and cross-country skiing. While most trails are off-limits to motor vehicles, some local trail organizations do allow ATVs and snowmobiles.

Trail descriptions themselves suggest an ideal itinerary for each route, including the best parking areas and access points, where to begin, your direction of travel, and any highlights along the way. The text notes any connecting or neighboring routes, with page numbers for the respective trail descriptions. Following each description are directions to the recommended trailheads.

Each trail description also lists a local contact (name, address, phone number, and Web site) for further information. Be sure to call these trail managers or volunteer groups in advance for updates and current conditions.

Key to Map Icons

Parking

Drinking water

Bathrooms

Trail Use

Rail-trails are popular routes for a range of uses, often making them busy places to play. Trail etiquette applies. If passing other trail users on your bicycle, always try to pass on the left with an audible warning such as a bike-mounted bell or a polite but firm, "Passing on your left!" For your safety and that of other trail users, keep children and pets from straying into oncoming trail traffic. Keep dogs leashed, and supervise children until they can demonstrate proper behavior.

Cyclists and inline skaters should wear helmets, reflective clothing, and other safety gear, as some trails involve hazardous road crossings. It's also best to bring a flashlight or bike- or helmet-mounted light for tunnel passages or twilight excursions.

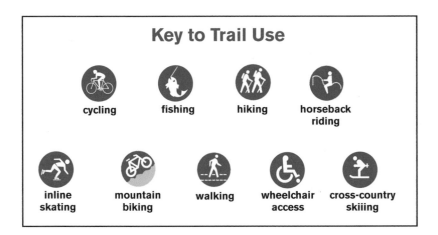

Learn More

While *Rail-Trails: Southeast* is a helpful guide to available routes in the region, it wasn't feasible to list every rail-trail in the Southeast, and new rail-trails spring up each year. To learn about additional rail-trails in your area or to plan a trip to an area beyond the scope of this book, log on to the Rails-to-Trails Conservancy home page (www.railstotrails. org) and click on the Find a Trail link. RTC's online database lists more than 1,400 rail-trails nationwide, searchable by state, county, city, trail name, surface type, length, activity, and/or keywords regarding your interest. A number of listings include photos and reviews from people who've already visited the trail.

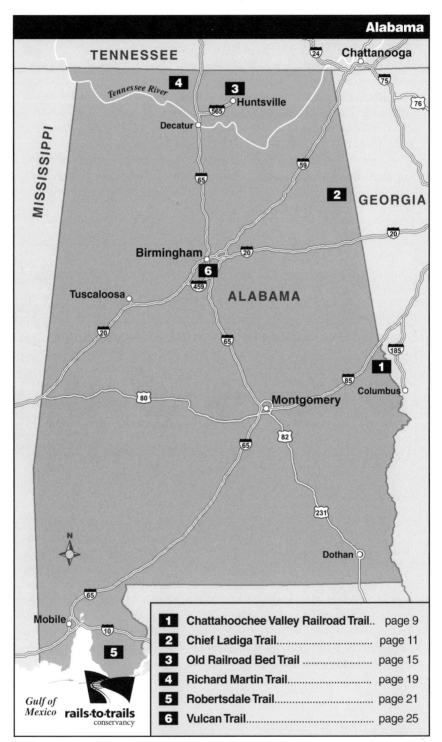

Alabama

TENNESSEE

Chattanooga

Tennessee River

Huntsville

Decatur

MISSISSIPPI

GEORGIA

Birmingham

Tuscaloosa

ALABAMA

Montgomery

Columbus

Dothan

N

Mobile

Gulf of Mexico

rails·to·trails
conservancy

Alabama

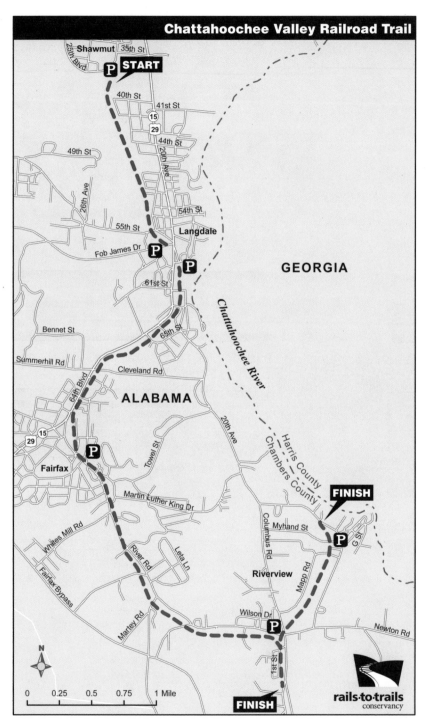

Chattahoochee Valley Railroad Trail

Shawmut 25th St 35th St
25th Blvd
P START
40th St
41st St
15
29
44th St
20th Ave
49th St
26th Ave
54th St
55th St Langdale
Fob James Dr **P**
P
61st St
GEORGIA
Bennet St
65th St
Summerhill Rd
Cleveland Rd
64th Blvd
Chattahoochee River
ALABAMA
15
29
20th Ave
P
Fairfax
Towel St
Martin Luther King Dr
Harris County
Chambers County
FINISH
Columbus Rd
Myhand St
P
Whites Mill Rd
River Rd
Leta Ln
Riverview
Mapp Rd
GA 18
Fairfax Bypass
Wilson Dr
Newton Rd
P
Martey Rd
1st St
N
0 0.25 0.5 0.75 1 Mile
FINISH
rails·to·trails
conservancy

Chattahoochee Valley Railroad Trail

On Alabama's eastern border, nestled amid gentle hills that overlook the mighty Chattahoochee River is a cluster of four small textile mill towns—Shawmut, Langdale, Fairfax, and Riverview—all on the National Registry of Historic Places. In 1980 these villages incorporated as the city of Valley, a community of nearly 10,000 residents.

The Chattahoochee Valley Railroad served the region for nearly 100 years, carrying passengers, cotton, cloth, and supplies. But the trains stopped running in 1992, and in 2000 this corridor became a rail-trail that winds past the communities and historical sites.

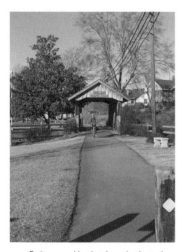

Built on an old railroad trestle, the trail passes through the Horace King Memorial Bridge in Valley.

The route begins in Shawmut along straight, quiet spans through tall pines, passing a few homes set back from the trail. Two miles along, in Langdale, the trail stops just shy of moderately busy, two-lane US Highway 29. Cross the road here and pick up the trail again a block south. Or consider a short side trip to the Chattahoochee by heading east on 59th Street and taking an access road to the riverfront. You'll be rewarded with a stunning view of the river and may even spot a bald eagle.

Back on the trail, you'll pass several historic properties and bridges—most notable is the Langdale Mill, off the east side of the trail. Plans are underway to house shops and a conference center in the mill, which was originally built to stimulate the local economy following the Civil War.

Endpoints
Shawmut to Riverview

Mileage
7

Roughness Index
1

Surface
Asphalt

Continuing south, the trail parallels local roads, passing the 1917 Fairfax Depot, today a museum with welcome restrooms. Columbus Road marks a short trail extension to the south, but to finish the last mile of the trail, you'll follow the sharp turn north toward the river, passing through fragrant pines to Riverview.

DIRECTIONS

From I-85, take Exit 77 in Valley. Turn east on Fob James Drive and follow it to Langdale, then turn left on US Highway 29/20th Avenue. Continue about two miles until you pass a Wal-Mart on your left. At the next light, turn left on 35th Street, then left on 22nd Street. Parking for the trail's Shawmut access point is at road's end.

Contact: City of Valley Parks & Recreation Department
P.O. Box 186
Valley, AL 36854
(334) 756-5281

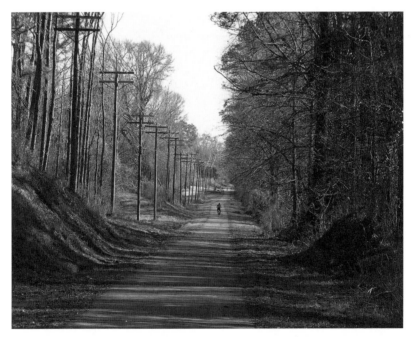

A relatively new rail-trail, the Chattahoochee Valley Railroad Trail was opened in 2000 and has since been embraced by locals for its town-to-town connections.

Chief Ladiga Trail

In northeast Alabama, the nearly 33-mile Chief Ladiga Trail is a regional playground that passes through welcoming towns and pastoral landscapes. Following a former CSX railroad corridor, the rail-trail is named for the Creek Indian leader who signed the 1832 Cusseta Treaty, surrendering the tribe's remaining land in the area.

Remarkably flat and mostly smooth (21.5 miles are paved; the remaining miles are gravel), the trails arcs from Woodland Park in Anniston northeast through small towns and quiet countryside to the state line. It begins on a slightly raised rail bed and then enters open fields, passing beneath canopies of pine, dogwood, and other native trees and alongside enchanting wetlands. You'll find numerous access points along the way.

The first stop is Weaver, where you might want to pop into the nearby grocery store for snacks. Back on the trail, twin stone foundations of a railroad trestle flank the route. Five miles along, in Jacksonville, you'll pass a train depot awaiting restoration and the Jacksonville State University campus. Just off the trail is the historic

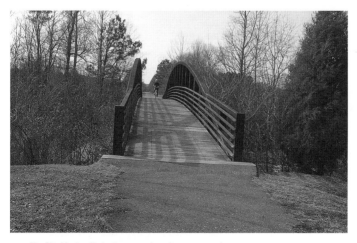

The Chief Ladiga Trail takes a gentle and scenic route between towns.

Endpoints
Anniston to Alabama/Georgia state line

Mileage
33

Roughness Index
1

Surface
Asphalt, gravel, dirt

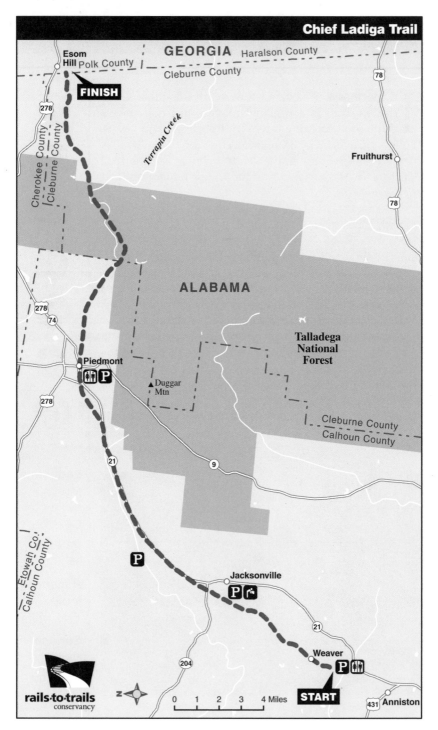

Chief Ladiga Trail

town square, which boasts several shops and restaurants (climb Mountain Street and turn right on Route 21).

Keep alert over the following nine miles, as you may catch a deer or fox watching you. You'll soon reach central Piedmont, a quaint community that embraces the trail with a welcome center, benches, and a sandwich shop just steps away.

From Piedmont the scenery begins to change. Duggar Mountain and the southern Appalachians provide a backdrop to fields that transition to forests. Terrapin Creek skirts the trail, and soon a bridge carries you over it. Here, the asphalt gives way to a rugged gravel trail through protected wilderness within Talladega National Forest. While inline skaters and cyclists must turn back here, the next 10 miles offer a continuing adventure for hikers, mountain bikers, and equestrians.

DIRECTIONS

From I-20, take Exit 185 and head north about 10 miles through Anniston on Route 1/Quintard Avenue, then bear right on McClellan Boulevard/Route 21 on the north side of town. A few miles past the split, turn left on Weaver Road, continue about a mile and a half, and then turn left again on Holly Farms Road to the well-marked Woodland Park trailhead.

Contact: Jacksonville State University
Environmental Policy & Information Center
700 Pelham Road North, Suite 246
Jacksonville, AL 36265
(256) 782-5681
http://epic.jsu.edu/clt/

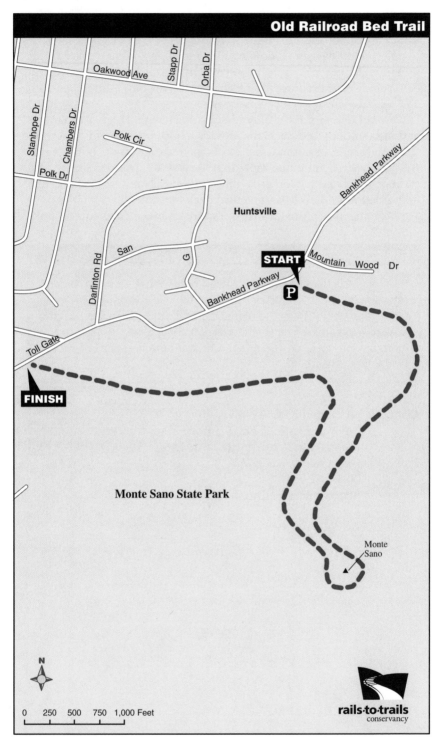

Old Railroad Bed Trail

Old Railroad Bed Trail

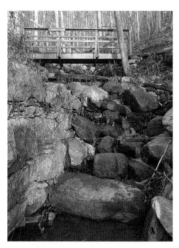

Foot bridges ease the crossing of brooks along the trail.

Boasting an intriguing history, the Old Railroad Bed Trail (a.k.a. Monte Sano Railroad Trail) follows one of the country's oldest and shortest-lived rail corridors. In the late 1800s, as yellow fever raged in Atlanta, a hotel was built atop 1,600-foot Monte Sano (which means "mountain of health" in Italian). Guests were drawn to the resort by the area's fresh springs, cool climates, and valley views. The rail line was built to ferry passengers from Huntsville, replacing the previous four-hour horse-and-carriage ride.

A construction crew of 500 men took just four months to complete the line, which included 8.5 miles of rail, five trestles, and four small bridges. (Earning a mere dollar for each 12-hour shift, these workers later staged Huntsville's first labor strike, demanding, without success, a 10-hour day.) The line opened in August 1888, but by October a derailment, caused by brake failure, had frightened passengers away. Afterward, only freight cars plied the line until the trains stopped running in 1896.

Launched in 1990, the Old Railroad Bed Trail was among the country's first rail-to-trail conversions. The Land Trust of Huntsville & North Alabama purchased the line, built the trail, and maintains it today. Those who stroll the narrow dirt and stone bed will pass cascading springs and the original stone bridge supports, built without mortar. Atop the peak, picture the Hotel Monte Sano, an elaborate, 223-room haven from turn-of-the-century health scares. Following your hike, head down to the Huntsville Depot Museum or the North Alabama Railroad Museum for more local railroad lore.

Endpoints
Bankhead Parkway
to Monte Sano
State Park,
Huntsville

Mileage
2

Roughness Index
3

Surface
Crushed stone, dirt

DIRECTIONS

From Huntsville, take Bankhead Parkway north to the Monte Sano State Park trailhead, which lies on the right a half-mile past the Toll Gate Road intersection. A stone marker stands at the entrance.

Contact: The Land Trust of Huntsville & North Alabama
907 Franklin Street
Huntsville, AL 35801
(256) 534-5263
www.landtrust-hsv.org/monte_sano_preserve.htm

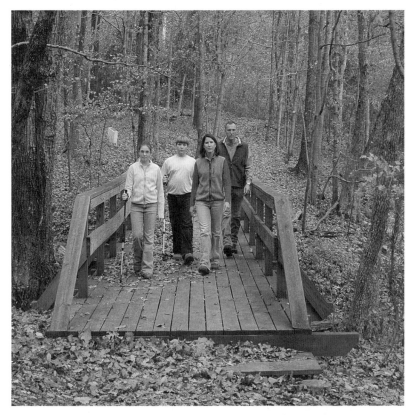

Golden and russet autumn leaves blanket the Old Railroad Bed Trail in Monte Sano State Park.

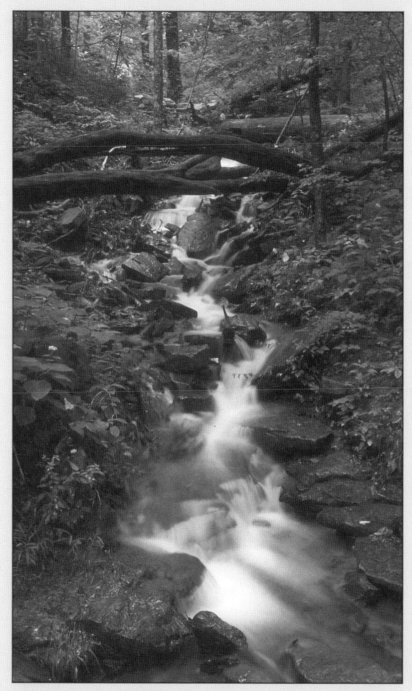

Spring rains swell creeks running through Monte Sano State Park.

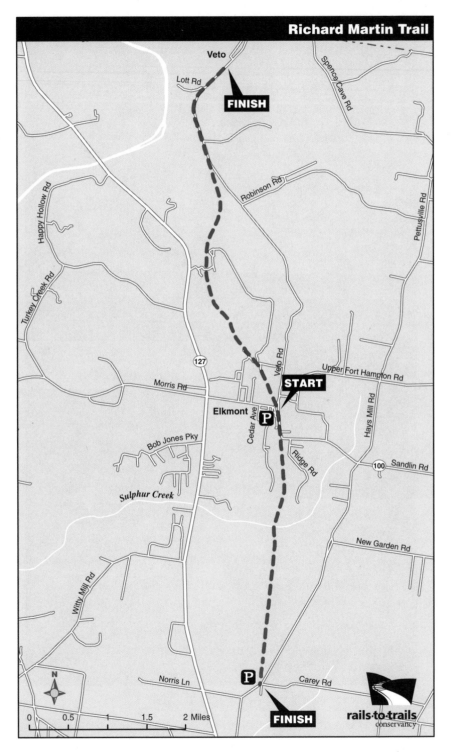

Richard Martin Trail

Richard Martin Trail

The Richard Martin Trail (a.k.a. Limestone Rail-Trail) is best accessed mid-route from a trailhead in the town of Elkmont, where you'll find parking, good signage, a historic depot (used for community activities), a refurbished railcar, a place to eat and antiques to acquire. You'll likely encounter horses along the trail, which is a favorite among equestrians. If you intend to bike the route, take a mountain bike or hybrid, as the rough terrain will give you—and your tires—a workout. Also be sure to bring food and drink, as Elkmont is the only place to purchase refreshments along the trail.

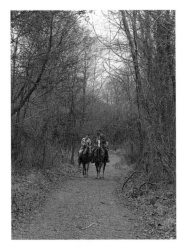

The Richard Martin Trail is enjoyed by equestrians, bicyclists, and walkers alike.

From town the trail heads both north and south, about four miles in either direction. To the north lie cotton fields, historic homesteads, and several new bridges. Over the first mile, the trail merges with local roads before establishing its independence. At present, the trail ends near the town of Veto.

The four miles of trail to the south offer different terrain, views, and history. Passing through pristine wetlands, you'll soon reach a slight incline, a mile south of Elkmont, where a trestle once spanned Sulphur Creek, the site of Alabama's bloodiest Civil War conflict. A plaque commemorates the 1864 Battle of Sulphur Creek Trestle, during which a Tennessee & Alabama Central Railroad supply train moving Union Army troops and goods from Nashville to Atlanta came under attack. More than 200 soldiers were killed during the ensuing firefight.

Endpoints
Veto to Hays Mill

Mileage
8

Roughness Index
2

Surface
Crushed stone, gravel

Until it was abandoned in 1986, the line brought in mail and supplies to area communities and brought out cotton, a mainstay of the local economy. The trail is named for local advocate Richard Martin, who continues to rally for the improvement and extension of the trail.

DIRECTIONS

From I-65, take Exit 361 and head west four miles on Sandlin Road/Route 100 toward Elkmont. The trailhead lies is on the left, marked by a restored depot and railcar.

Contact: City of Elkmont
(256) 732-4211

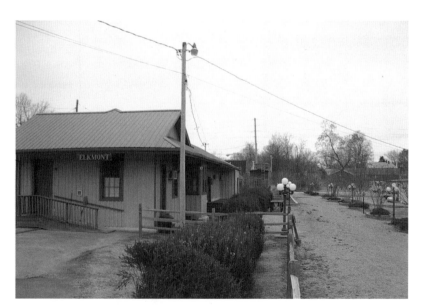

The historic Elkmont railroad depot hosts a restored railway car so that visitors may get a taste of the trail's railroad past.

Robertsdale Trail

T he Robertsdale Trail (a.k.a. Central Baldwin Rail-Trail) is a short linear route through the heart of Robertsdale along a former Louisville & Nashville Railroad line. While you won't find a formal trailhead facility or parking area, secure public parking is available at the main post office near the trail's northern terminus, on US Highway 90 about a mile from the charming southern downtown. The city police department and county sheriff's office stand nearby.

The trail is generally wide enough to accommodate its variety of users, though at several road crossings it narrows to a concrete sidewalk. At other points the trail splits, allowing users to move in opposite directions. Along these sections, trailside benches, landscaping, and mature southern flora draw small gatherings of locals, lending to the trail's small-town feeling and sense of community. Pause for a meal or browse the shops in downtown Robertsdale during your return stroll through this delightful town.

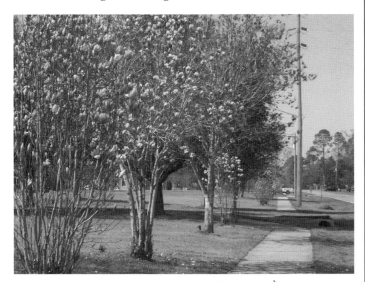

Magnolia trees bloom freely beside the Robertsdale Trail in early spring.

Endpoints
Hughen Street to East Silverhill Avenue, Robertsdale

Mileage
2

Roughness Index
1

Surface
Asphalt

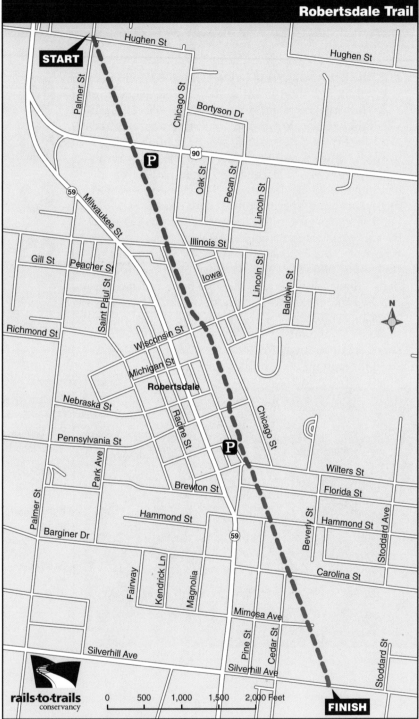

Robertsdale Trail

START

Hughen St

Hughen St

Palmer St

Chicago St

Bortyson Dr

90

59

Milwaukee St

Oak St

Pecan St

Lincoln St

Gill St

Peacher St

Saint Paul St

Illinois St

Lincoln St

Iowa

Baldwin St

Richmond St

Wisconsin St

Michigan St

Robertsdale

Nebraska St

Racine St

Chicago St

Pennsylvania St

Park Ave

Wilters St

Florida St

Palmer St

Brewton St

Beverly St

Stoddard Ave

Barginer Dr

Hammond St

Hammond St

59

Carolina St

Fairway

Kendrick Ln

Magnolia

Mimosa Ave

Pine St

Cedar St

Stoddard St

Silverhill Ave

Silverhill Ave

rails·to·trails
conservancy

0   500   1,000   1,500   2,000 Feet

FINISH

DIRECTIONS

Take I-10 to Route 59 south into Robertsdale, then turn east on US Highway 90. The post office is on the left, just past the trail crossing. Cyclists and walkers can access the trail from here as well as from its southern terminus on East Silverhill Avenue.

Contact: City of Robertsdale
Department of Public Works
22650 East Chicago Street
Robertsdale, AL 36567
(251) 947-8950
www.robertsdale.org/publicworks/index.html

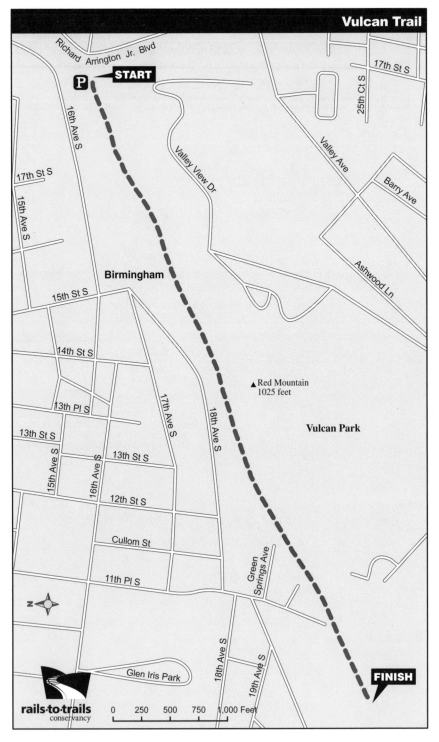

Vulcan Trail

Richard Arrington Jr. Blvd

P START

16th Ave S

17th St S

25th Ct S

17th St S

15th Ave S

Valley View Dr

Valley Ave

Barry Ave

Ashwood Ln

Birmingham

15th St S

14th St S

13th Pl S

17th Ave S

18th Ave S

▲ Red Mountain
1025 feet

Vulcan Park

13th St S

15th Ave S

16th Ave S

13th St S

12th St S

Cullom St

Green Springs Ave

11th Pl S

N

Glen Iris Park

18th Ave S

19th Ave S

FINISH

rails·to·trails
conservancy

0   250   500   750   1,000 Feet

Vulcan Trail

Birmingham's mile-long Vulcan Trail scales the ridge of 1,025-foot Red Mountain. In summer, the tree-lined trail offers cool respite from the heat, while bare winter trees yield city views. Best of all, it takes little effort to enjoy this breathtaking scenery; like most rail-trails, the route is flat.

The paved surface is especially inviting for walkers, joggers, and those taking pets for a stroll. From the parking area, the path traces the route of the former L&N Birmingham Mineral Railroad. (With roots as a steel town, Birmingham is one of the few geologic zones where one can find all three mineral components—iron ore, coal, and limestone—needed to make steel.)

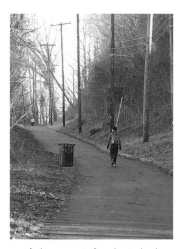

A pleasant respite from the city bustle awaits you on the Vulcan Trail.

The trail offers a bird's-eye view of many notable historic structures and areas, including the Arlington Antebellum Home and the Birmingham Civil Rights District, a six-block tribute to the civil rights movement that contains the Alabama Jazz Hall of Fame and the Sixteenth Street Baptist Church, site of an infamous 1963 Ku Klux Klan bombing that killed four young black girls.

The route runs below 10-acre Vulcan Park, home to the world's largest cast-iron statue and trail/park namesake. Italian sculptor Giuseppe Moretti crafted the 56-foot statue of Vulcan, the Roman god of fire, for the 1904 World's Fair in St. Louis, to showcase Birmingham's burgeoning industrial might. The park also houses the Vulcan Center, which traces the city's industrial past and offers rotating exhibits. While the park remains inaccessible from the trail, plans call for that to change.

Endpoints
Richard Arrington Boulevard (near Vulcan Park) to 11th Place South, Birmingham

Mileage
1

Roughness Index
1

Surface
Asphalt

DIRECTONS

From I-65, take Exit 256-A/Oxmoor Road and drive east about a mile toward Homewood; Oxmoor becomes Palisades Boulevard. Turn right on Valley Avenue, drive 1.6 miles, then turn left on Richard Arrington Jr. Boulevard. The trailhead is 0.2 mile down on the left.

Contact: Vulcan Park Foundation
1701 Valley View Drive
Birmingham, AL 35209
(205) 933-1409
www.vulcanpark.org

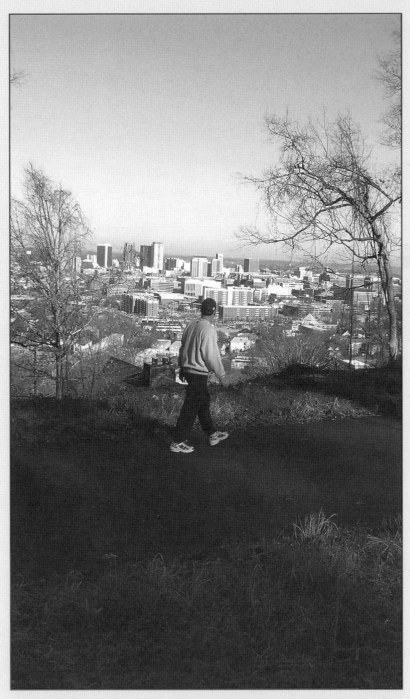

Catch some great views of Birmingham through the trees as you stretch your legs on the short Vulcan Trail.

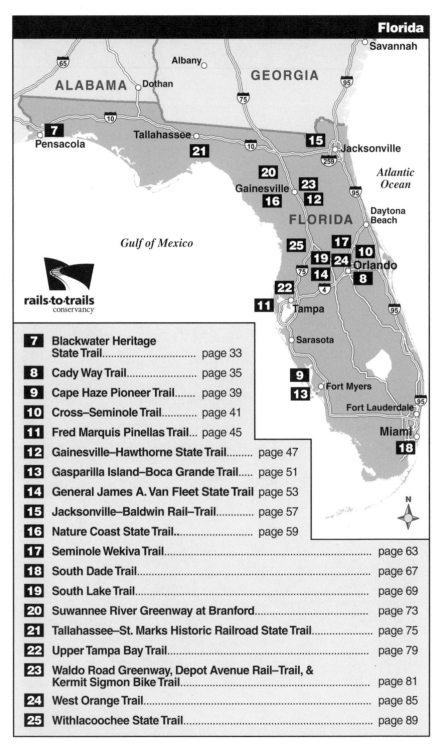

Florida

Savannah

Albany

ALABAMA Dothan

GEORGIA

Pensacola

Tallahassee

Jacksonville

Atlantic
Ocean

Gainesville

Daytona
Beach

FLORIDA

Gulf of Mexico

Orlando

Tampa

Sarasota

Fort Myers

Fort Lauderdale

Miami

rails·to·trails
conservancy

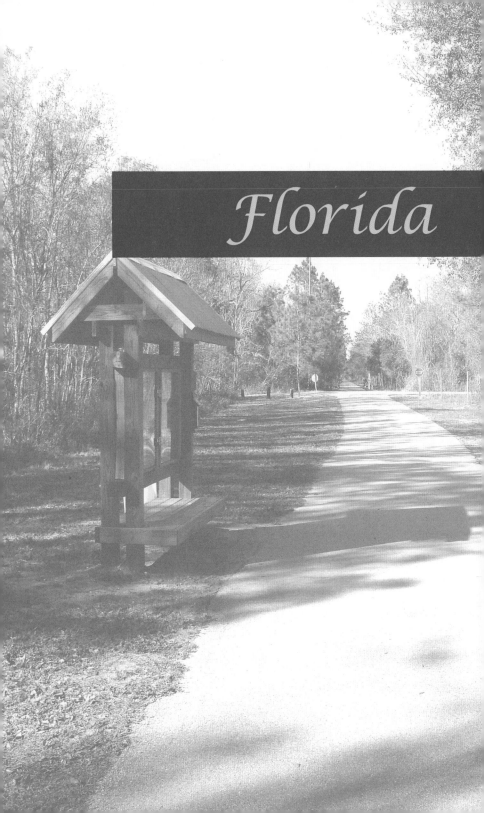

Florida

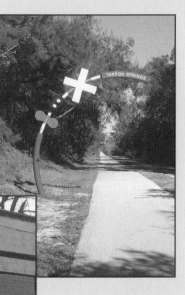

A Tarpon Spring trail marker
on the Fred Marquis Pinellas trail

Trailside mural on the Nature Coast
State Trail

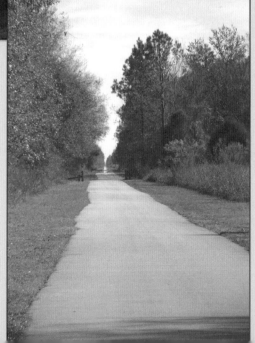

A long, straight stretch on the General
James A. Van Fleet State Trail

FLORIDA KEYS OVERSEAS HERITAGE TRAIL

The sections listed below are part of a 106.5-mile trail that will run the length of the Florida Keys along Henry Flagler's old railroad line. It will cross many of the original railroad bridges subsequently converted for automobile use in the 1950s. Some of these have been converted back to their original configuration, but with added safety rails and an asphalt surface. To accommodate fishing, platforms will be added to some of the reconditioned spans, including the 2.2-mile Long Key Bridge and smaller spans at Toms Harbor and Toms Harbor Cut. Bear in mind that this multimillion-dollar project is a complex, long-term undertaking and remains far from complete. Trail sections often begin or end at roadways or bridges with inadequate shoulders, causing potentially dangerous traffic encounters. In 2005, Hurricane Katrina set things back further by damaging and/or washing away several sections. The stretch at Saddlebunch Key, in particular, will be missed until repaired.

Sections worth visiting include:

- Lower Matacombe, 4.4 miles (Mile Marker 74–MM 77)
- Long Key Bridge, 2.2 miles (Mile Marker 65–MM 67)
- Grassy Key, 4 miles (Mile Marker 54.5–MM 58.5)
- Toms Harbor/Toms Harbor Cut, 5 miles (Mile Marker 54.5–MM 59.5)

Contact: Florida Keys Overseas Heritage Trail
Office of Greenways & Trails
3 La Croix Court
Key Largo, FL 33037
(305) 853-3571

Endpoints
Key Largo
(Mile Marker 106.5) to
Key West
(Mile Marker 0)

Mileage
106.5

Roughness Index
3

Surface
Nonexistent to asphalt

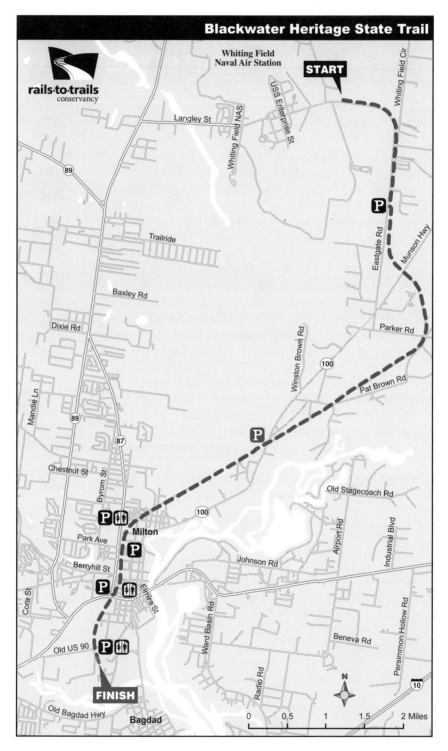

Blackwater Heritage State Trail

Blackwater Heritage State Trail

In Milton, just northeast of Pensacola, the 10-mile Blackwater Heritage State Trail is the rewarding result of a partnership between Florida's Departments of Transportation and Environmental Protection and the US Navy. Its northernmost mile and a half is officially dubbed the Military Heritage Trail.

Five convenient trailheads provide access, while a smooth asphalt surface promises an enjoyable ride through flat rural and urban areas. The Milton trailhead offers parking and restroom facilities, nearby restaurants, and even a bicycle shop for last-minute gear and supplies.

A mile up the trail, local citizens staff a visitor center and provide information about this and other area parks and attractions. As the route streaks north, the surroundings become increasingly rural. Telltale signs that you're leaving Milton behind include trailside pitcher plants and rabbit sightings.

By the time you reach the Munson Highway parking area, just under three miles along the trail, the rural setting dominates. Munson provides the only horse trailer parking, so expect to spot more equestrians on the adjacent trail and at the seven nearby shared stream crossings.

Endpoints
Milton to the Whiting Field Naval Air Station

Mileage
10

Roughness Index
1

Surface
Asphalt

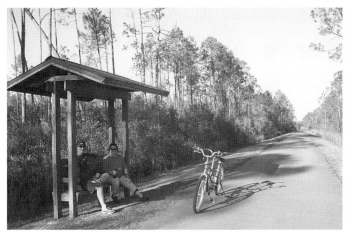

Rest areas along the trail make this a pleasant place for trail users of all ages and abilities.

Large stands of windblown trees that lean at 45-degree angles speak to past hurricanes.

The trail ends abruptly at the gates of the Whiting Field Naval Air Station. Prior to September 2001, the trail continued west to an active airport runway, but national and local security precautions now prevent that. **Shutterbugs take note:** While the military embraces the trail, security officers at the base entrance may be uncomfortable with you snapping pictures of this area.

DIRECTIONS

From I-10, take Route 87 toward Milton. The trailhead is on the northwest corner of the Route 87/US Highway 90 intersection. The trailside visitor center is at 5533 Alabama Street, a mile north of the Milton trailhead. Parking is available.

To reach the Munson Highway parking area and its equestrian parking, head north from Milton about three miles on Route 191 to the trail intersection.

The Whiting Field trailhead is a few miles north of the Route 87A/Route 191 intersection, just northeast of Milton.

Contact: Blackwater Heritage State Trail
5533 Alabama Street
Milton, FL 32564
(850) 983-5338
www.dep.state.fl.us/gwt/guide/regions/panhandlewest/
trails/black_heritage.htm

Cady Way Trail

Winding its way through northeast Orlando, the Cady Way Trail passes through several urban neighborhoods and parks. It's broken into two sections, soon to be connected by a pedestrian bridge. The southern section of the trail is longer and attracts more people, while the northern section is new and less known.

The well-marked southern trailhead sits just off Herndon Avenue across from the Orlando Fashion Square Mall. From here the trail leads east about a mile, passing several busy intersections, but pedestrian safety is a high priority in Orlando, as evidenced by traffic lights built specifically for these crossings. The trail then swings north and follows the shore of Lake Baldwin for 2.5 miles. You'll eventually emerge in Cady Way Park, a lovely shaded park with a playground, basketball courts, picnic areas, and public restrooms.

A half mile from the park is the gap across Semoran Boulevard that the pedestrian bridge will eventually span. On the far side, the trail continues 1.5 miles north to Goldenrod Park, the best access point along this section.

Endpoints
Fashion Square Mall to Aloma Avenue and Howell Branch Road, Orlando

Mileage
6

Roughness Index
1

Surface
Asphalt

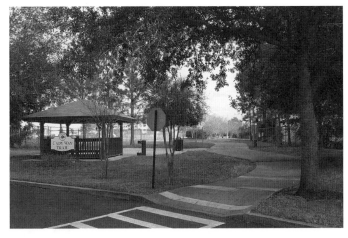

Pedestrian safety is paramount on the Cady Way Trail.

35

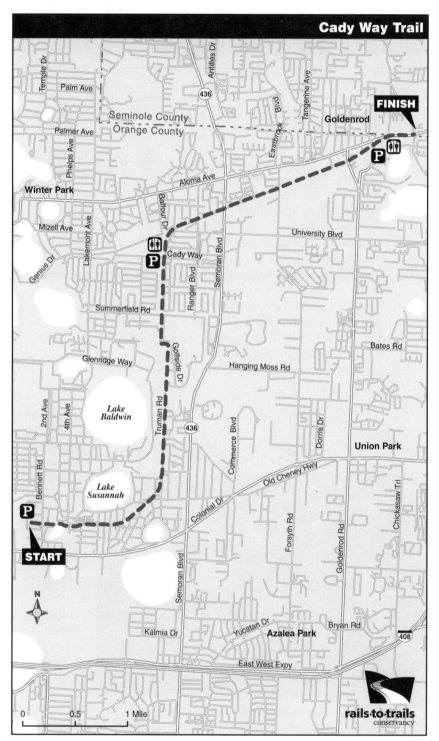

Cady Way Trail

The trail officially ends at the intersection of Aloma Avenue and Howell Branch Road, but you don't have to stop there, as access to 2.5 miles of the Cross-Seminole Trail (see page 41) lies on the opposite corner of the intersection.

DIRECTIONS

To reach the southern trailhead, take I-4 downtown to Route 50, then head east to Herndon Avenue (about 2.5 miles) and turn left. The trailhead is a half mile north, adjacent to the Fashion Square Mall and a post office.

To reach Cady Way Park, take Route 436 to Aloma Avenue, head west, then turn left on Ranger Boulevard and right on Cady Way. The park is four blocks ahead on the right.

To reach Goldenrod Park, take Route 436 to Aloma Avenue, head east about 1.6 miles and look for the park sign on the right.

Contact: Orange County Parks & Recreation Department
4801 West Colonial Drive
Orlando, FL 32808
(407) 836-6160
www.orangecountyfl.net/dept/cesrvcs/parks/default.asp

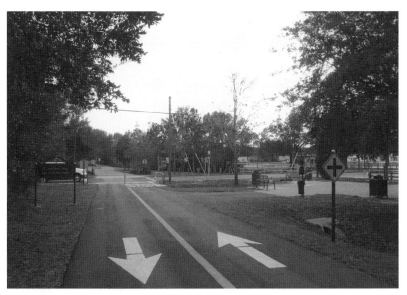

Clear signage and safe street crossings make for a smooth ride on the Cady Way Trail.

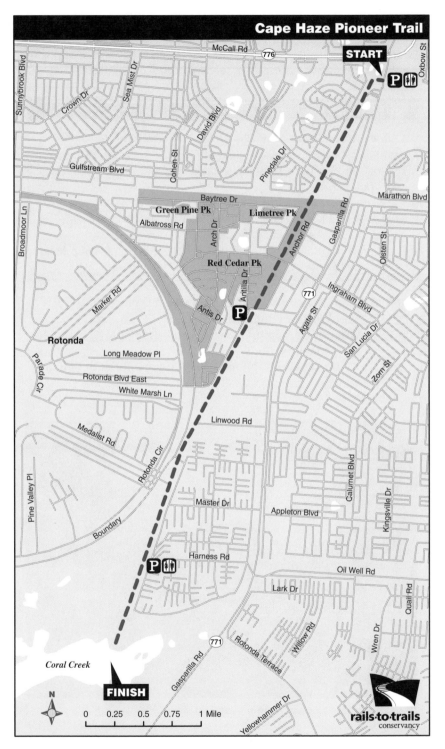

Cape Haze Pioneer Trail

When you walk, run, skate or bike the 5.5-mile Cape Haze Pioneer Trail, you're tracing the line that once serviced Florida's early phosphate industry and also moved people, livestock, and locally grown crops such as watermelons to waiting steamships in Boca Grande on Gasparilla Island. The long-running Charlotte Harbor & Northern Railroad operated until the late 1970s. Today there are plans to extend the trail south to the gulf and connect it with the Boca Grande Bike Path on Gasparilla Island, which shares the corridor. The resulting regional trail will span coastal Charlotte and Lee counties.

The fairly straight and flat rail-trail offers a relaxing ride and welcome relief from the area's growing traffic congestion. From its origins near Charlotte Beach, the trail has a rural feel, while multiple access points offer a break whenever you need one. Boasting ample parking, water, and restroom facilities, the northern trailhead is named after longtime trail advocates Dr. Robert and Anne Mercer, credited with starting Charlotte County's thriving rail-trail movement.

Endpoints
McCall (State
Road 776 and
State Road 771)
to Harness Road,
Rotonda

Mileage
5.5

**Roughness
Index**
1

Surface
Asphalt

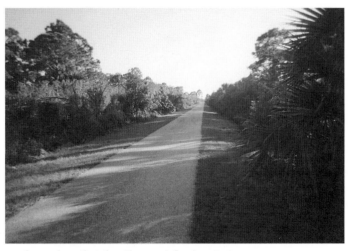

A sunny day on the trail provides an oasis from busy streets.

A quarter-mile beyond the Harness Road access point, named for trail advocate R. David Johnson, the trail ends at Coral Creek. The vaunted extension is in the works, however. A new housing development has already incorporated the trail into its layout, and a commercial development on the northern end built an extension leading to its tenants.

DIRECTIONS

To reach the Dr. Robert and Anne Mercer Trailhead from Port Charlotte, take Route 776 west to Route 771 south. The trailhead lies on the right about a block south of the intersection.

To reach the Rotonda Boulevard East trailhead, follow the above directions, but continue south on Route 771 about two miles, then turn right on Rotonda. The trailhead is on the left.

To reach the R. David Johnson Trailhead, follow the directions to the Rotonda trailhead, but continue south on Route 771 just over two miles to Harness Road. Turn right on Harness and continue to the trailhead.

Contact: Charlotte County Parks & Recreation
4500 Harbor Blvd.
Port Charlotte, FL 33952
(941) 627-1628
www.charlottecountyfl.com/parks/parkpages/
capehaze.html

Cross-Seminole Trail

Stretching from Orlando's densely populated outskirts to the sleepy bedroom communities of Oviedo, Winter Springs, and Lake Mary, the Cross-Seminole Trail provides crucial residential links in this automobile-dominated region. Throughout the day you'll encounter locals using it to get around town or simply exercise. The trail comprises four separate sections that will eventually connect to create an impressive 23-mile continuous trail. These open sections total some 14 miles and connect to other area rail-trails: the 14-mile Seminole Wekiva Trail to the west (see page 63) and the six-mile Cady Way Trail to the south (see page 35).

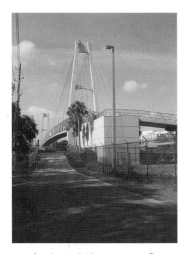

A pedestrian bridge crosses over Route 434 on the Cross-Seminole Trail.

The 2.8-mile southern section starts on the northeast corner of the Aloma Avenue/Howell Branch Road intersection, on the Seminole/Orange county line. (Signs for the Cady Way Trail mark the opposite corner.) This section follows Aloma Avenue northeast though a largely urban setting, coming to an abrupt end in a wooded area about 200 yards from the road.

The second section extends northwest from downtown Oviedo to Winter Springs. From the intersection of Railroad Street and North Central Avenue, you'll enter a pleasant wooded area and wend through several quiet, upscale neighborhoods. After 3.5 miles you'll reach the Black Hammock Trailhead, which offers the only sufficient parking along this section. At trail's end a beautifully constructed concrete pedestrian bridge crosses Route 434. Unfortunately, once you reach the woods on the far side, you have no choice but to turn back.

Endpoints
Seminole/Orange county line to Lake Mary

Mileage
14

Roughness Index
1

Surface
Asphalt

41

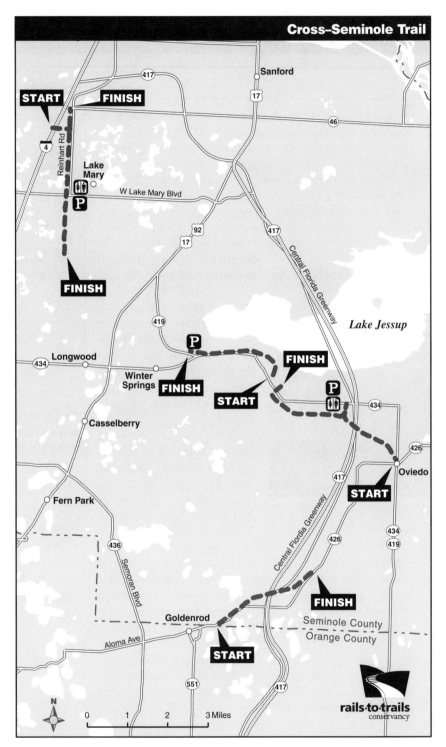

Cross–Seminole Trail

START FINISH

Reinhart Rd

4

Lake Mary

W Lake Mary Blvd

P

FINISH

92

17

419

Longwood
434

Winter Springs

FINISH

Casselberry

Fern Park

436

Semoran Blvd

Goldenrod

Aloma Ave

551

417

Sanford

17

46

417

Central Flordia Greenway

Lake Jessup

P

FINISH

START

P

434

426

Oviedo

417

START

434
419

426

Central Flordia Greenway

FINISH

Seminole County
Orange County

START

N

0   1   2   3 Miles

rails·to·trails
conservancy

The next section begins some 2,000 feet away, just through the woods. There are plans to connect the trails, though parking is currently insufficient. For now, the drive to reach the trailhead is worth the effort. From Layer Elementary School in Winter Springs, this pleasant 2.5-mile stretch passes behind Winter Springs High School and threads through peaceful neighborhoods.

The final four-mile section of the Cross-Seminole is quite different from the other three. The largely urban path parallels busy Reinhart Road in Lake Mary for much of its length. Headed south from Route 46A to Greenwood Boulevard, you'll follow a bustling business corridor with many road crossings. If you need a break from high-volume traffic once you reach trail's end, simply hop on the connecting spur to the Seminole Wekiva Trail (see page 63), on the west side of Reinhardt Road at the Oakland Hills Circle intersection.

DIRECTIONS FROM DOWNTOWN ORLANDO

To reach the Aloma Avenue trailhead, take Route 436 to Aloma, drive east about 1.6 miles, and look for the park sign on the right.

To reach the Black Hammock trailhead, take Route 408 east to the Central Florida Greeneway and head north toward Oviedo/Winter Springs. Exit at westbound Route 434/Sanford Oviedo Road and take the first left into the well-marked parking lot.

To reach the Layer Elementary School trailhead, follow the above directions to Black Hammock, but continue west another four miles on Route 434/Sanford Oviedo Road. Turn right on Route 419, then right again at Layer Elementary School. The trail will be on your right.

To reach the Lake Mary trailhead, take I-4 east to the Lake Mary Boulevard exit. Head east on Lake Mary about a mile to Reinhart Road; the trailhead is on the northeast corner.

Contact: Seminole County Trails & Greenways
520 West Lake Mary Blvd., Suite 200
Sanford, FL 32773
(407) 665-2093
www.seminolecountyfl.gov/pw/trails/trails_crosssem.asp

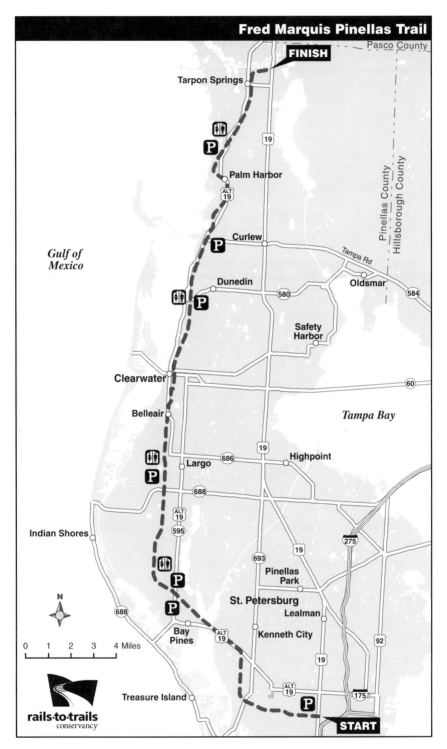

Fred Marquis Pinellas Trail

Pasco County

FINISH

Tarpon Springs

19

Palm Harbor

ALT
19

Curlew

*Gulf of
Mexico*

Dunedin

580

Oldsmar

584

Tampa Rd

Pinellas County
Hillsborough County

Safety
Harbor

Clearwater

60

Belleair

Tampa Bay

686

19

Highpoint

Largo

688

ALT
19

595

Indian Shores

693

19

275

Pinellas
Park

N

St. Petersburg

Lealman

0 1 2 3 4 Miles

688

Bay
Pines

ALT
19

Kenneth City

92

19

rails·to·trails
conservancy

Treasure Island

ALT
19

175

START

Fred Marquis Pinellas Trail

One of Florida's most popular and unique urban pathways, the Pinellas Trail spans the 34 miles from St. Petersburg north to Tarpon Springs, connecting several county parks, coastal areas, and communities. Its multiple access points, mile markers, and parking areas make the trail—and the communities it connects—very popular destinations among cyclists.

Over the first 15 miles from St. Petersburg, the trail crosses dozens of pedestrian bridges with sweeping views of the urban landscape. The most scenic of these is the quarter-mile Cross Bayou Bridge, which spans Boca Ciega Bay.

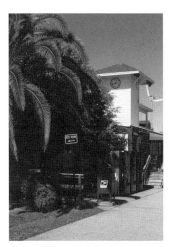

The Fred Marquis Pinellas Trail gets more than 1 million visitors a year.

Farther north lie the towns of Largo, Clearwater, and Dunedin. Pay close attention as you pass through downtown Clearwater because the trail merges with sidewalks and is not well marked. Dunedin offers a particularly pleasant scene, with shops, restaurants, public restrooms, and parking. The Gulf of Mexico is just two blocks away, worth the brief detour for lovely coastal scenery.

The final 10-mile stretch begins in the quiet township of Palm Harbor. Pause on the Bayshore Boulevard pedestrian bridge at Mile Marker 29 for more gulf scenery. The final few miles take you through Tarpon Springs' quaint business district. Trail's end is at Mile Marker 34 along US Highway 19; the trail extension just beyond the underpass to the east is not part of the Pinellas Trail.

Endpoints
St. Petersburg to Tarpon Springs

Mileage
34

Roughness Index
1

Surface
Asphalt

DIRECTIONS

The southern endpoint is in Trailhead Park on US Highway 19 in St. Petersburg, between Fairfield Avenue and Eighth Avenue South, while the northern endpoint is on US Highway 19 in Tarpon Springs, just south of the Anclote River.

There is no parking at either endpoint, but plenty of options line the route.

Contact: Pinellas County Planning Department
600 Cleveland Street, Suite 750
Clearwater, FL 33755
(727) 464-8201
www.pinellascounty.org/trailgd/default.htm

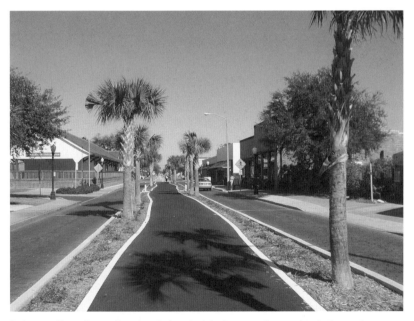

In downtown Tarpon Springs, the trail sits between brick-lined streets and passes through charming business districts.

Gainesville–Hawthorne State Trail

Connecting the university town of Gainesville with rural Hawthorne, this nearly 17-mile trail makes for a great day trip, complete with a thigh-burning hill or two and plenty of wildlife. While the path roughly parallels Route 20, it also traverses one of Florida's most environmentally sensitive areas: Paynes Prairie State Preserve. Just south of Gainesville, the park—though not the trail—is accessible via US Highway 441.

The well-maintained trail accommodates users with a 10-foot-wide paved path, regular trailheads and benches, and even a convenience store here and there. Between the Gainesville and Lochloosa trailheads, equestrians are given free rein on an adjacent grassy trail.

From its western endpoint in Gainesville's Boulware Springs Park, the trail soon leads to the Paynes Prairie overlook, and two miles from the trailhead you'll enter the preserve itself. This area boasted a thriving lake with routine steamboat activity until 1891, when a sinkhole drained the basin, leaving behind a mixed landscape of prairie, marsh, and open water.

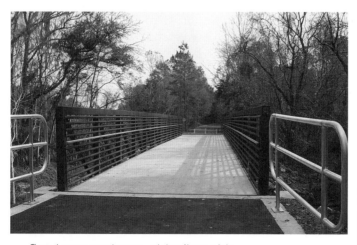

The trail crosses several streams and skirts Newnans Lake.

Endpoints
Gainesville to Hawthorne

Mileage
16.5

Roughness Index
1

Surface
Asphalt

47

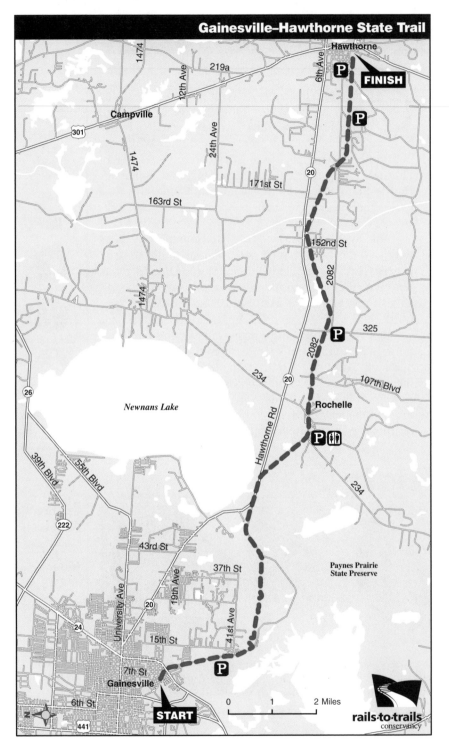

Gainesville–Hawthorne State Trail

Hawthorne

FINISH

Campville

219a

Newnans Lake

Rochelle

Paynes Prairie
State Preserve

Gainesville

START

0   1   2 Miles

rails·to·trails
conservancy

Several trailside overlooks offer views of the prairie, home to bison, wild horses, and numerous alligators. Park regulations ban visitors from feeding the gators, and dogs are not permitted, even if leashed. Rangers strictly enforce these rules. A half mile into the park, a side trip on the La Chua Trail leads to another viewing area; bicycles are not permitted on this unpaved spur.

Work is underway to extend the trail farther west into Gainesville to connect with the Waldo Road Greenway, Depot Avenue Rail-Trail, & Kermit Sigmon Bike Trail (see page 81).

DIRECTIONS

To reach the Boulware Springs Park trailhead from downtown Gainesville, take University Avenue east, fork right on Route 20, and take the next right on SE 15th Street. Boulware Springs Park (3500 SE 15th Street) is a couple of miles down on the right. Follow signs to the trail.

To reach the Lochloosa trailhead (7209 SE 200th Drive) from Hawthorne, take Route 2082 west, then turn left on SE 200th Drive. Park where the trail intersects the road.

To reach the Hawthorne trailhead (300 SW Second Avenue), take US Highway 301 south through Hawthorne and follow the brown signs along residential streets to the trailhead.

Contact: Gainesville–Hawthorne State Trail
3400 SE 15 Street
Gainesville, FL 32641
(352) 466-3397
www.floridastateparks.org/gainesville-hawthorne

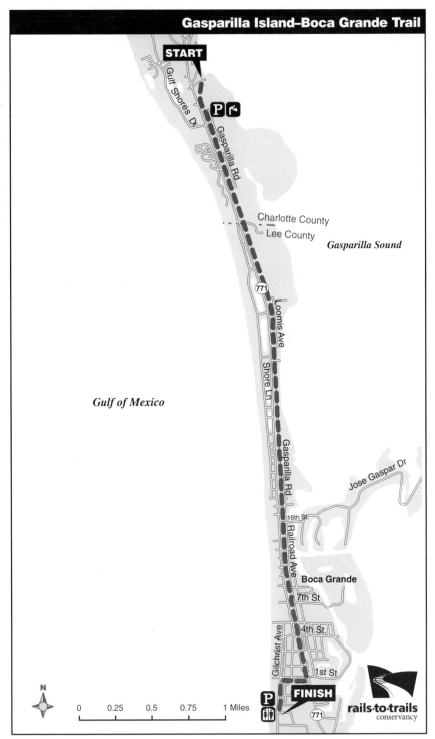

Gasparilla Island–Boca Grande Trail

START

Gulf Shores Dr

P

Gasparilla Rd

Charlotte County
Lee County

Gasparilla Sound

771

Loomis Ave

Shore Ln

Gulf of Mexico

Gasparilla Rd.

Jose Gaspar Dr

16th St.

Railroad Ave

Boca Grande

7th St

4th St.

Gilchrist Ave

1st St

P

FINISH

771

rails·to·trails
conservancy

N

0   0.25   0.5   0.75   1 Miles

Gasparilla Island– Boca Grande Trail

Visitors come to Gasparilla Island for its soothing beaches, upscale eateries, shopping, and the sense of history in and around Boca Grande, and you can sample it all along this paved 6.5-mile trail, known locally as the Boca Grande Bike Path. Credited as Florida's first rail-trail, the path travels the length of this Gulf Coast barrier island, offering a host of activities, from sunbathing to state park rambles. Remember to bring your sunscreen—and your wallet: While use of the trail is free, the causeway crossing and sites along the route charge fees.

If you start from the south shore, consider paying the state park entrance fee to visit the museum, which chronicles the island's history and fishing industry. Two miles north lies the Range Light Beach Access and its namesake squat historic lighthouse.

Those who start from the north will have their pick of beautiful Gasparilla Sound overlooks. Also watch for the nonnative iguanas that have successfully inhabited this lush, palm-covered island. This end offers a separate jogging track as well.

Endpoints
Gasparilla Island Causeway to Range Light Beach Access

Mileage
6.5

Roughness Index
1.5

Surface
Asphalt

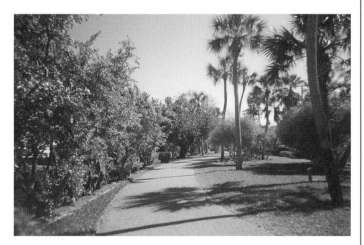

The Gasparilla Island–Boca Grande Trail treats you to numerous views of the Gulf of Mexico and Gasparilla Sound.

Whichever direction you choose, the beautifully landscaped and well-kept trail soon reaches central Boca Grande, just south of the trail midpoint. The old Boca Grande Depot has been converted into an upscale commercial center, and behind it lies a section of preserved track. Surprisingly, golf carts harmoniously share the trail with other users, showcasing a unique blend of Southern hospitality and practical transportation for residents and visitors alike.

DIRECTIONS

To access the northern trailhead from Port Charlotte, take Route 776 south to Route 771, which accesses the island via the Boca Grande Causeway (toll). The trailhead is on the left, just past the causeway.

To reach the Range Light Beach Access, follow the above directions onto the island, but continue on Route 771 south. The access point is on the right, within sight of the old lighthouse.

Contact: Gasparilla Island Conservation
& Improvement Association
P.O. Box 446
Boca Grande, FL 33921
(914) 964-2667
www.dep.state.fl.us/gwt/guide/regions/westcentral/
trails/gasparilla_island.htm

FLORIDA

General James A. Van Fleet State Trail

The General James A. Van Fleet State Trail runs 29 miles through some of Florida's most scenic rural landscape. If you are looking to immerse yourself in wetlands and wildlife, it will not disappoint; at least one-third of the trail crosses central Florida's 322,690-acre Green Swamp.

The trail stretches from Polk City north to the town of Mabel on Route 50. The Polk City trailhead offers ample parking, picnic, and restroom facilities, plus an expansive field of clipped grass, perfect for a game of pickup soccer.

The flat and arrow-straight route, with just one slight curve around Mile Marker 5, is a favorite among time-trial cyclists in the area; though thanks to its remote setting, you'll likely encounter only the occasional speedster.

The Green Pond Road trailhead, near Mile Marker 10, marks the boundary of the Green Swamp, one of Florida's protected wetland and wildlife areas. From here on watch for feral pigs, armadillos, buzzards, and possibly an alligator or two basking on the trail's warm asphalt surface.

Endpoints
Polk City to Mabel

Mileage
29

Roughness Index
2

Surface
Asphalt, gravel, dirt

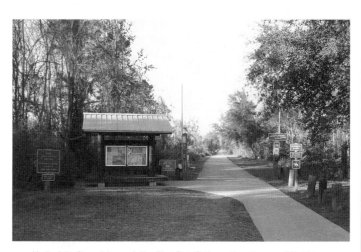
Much of the General James A. Van Fleet State Trail runs through some of Florida's beguiling swamps.

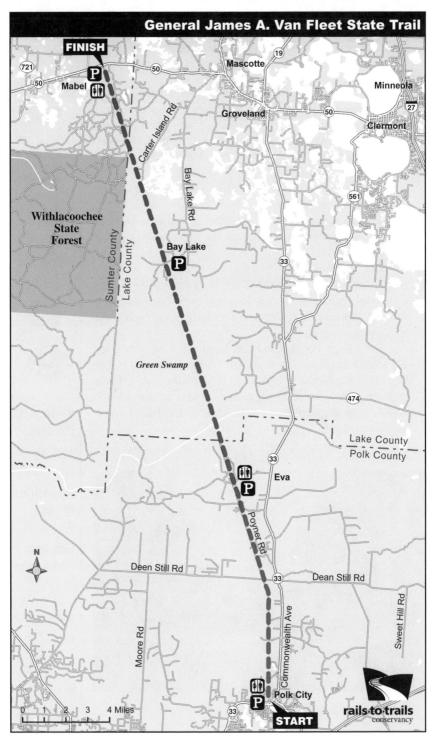

General James A. Van Fleet State Trail

FINISH

721

Mascotte

50

50

Mabel

Minneola

50

Groveland

Clermont

27

Carter Island Rd

561

Bay Lake Rd

Withlacoochee
State
Forest

Bay Lake

33

Sumter County

Lake County

Green Swamp

474

Lake County
Polk County

33

Eva

33

Poyner Rd

N

Deen Still Rd

Dean Still Rd

33

Sweet Hill Rd

Moore Rd

Commonwealth Ave

0 1 2 3 4 Miles

Polk City

33

START

rails·to·trails
conservancy

While the Bay Lake trailhead signals the end of the protected reserve, the final 10 miles of the Van Fleet State Trail to the Mabel trailhead are every bit as scenic. The decision is yours whether to race back to Polk City or savor the return trip along this beautiful, serene trail.

DIRECTIONS

To reach the Polk City trailhead from Lakeland, take I-4 east to Exit 38/Polk City and follow Route 33 north to Polk City. The trailhead is at the intersection of Route 33 and Route 655/Berkley Road.

To reach the Green Pond Road trailhead from Clermont, take Route 50 west to Route 33 south. Follow Route 33 about 16 miles to Green Pond Road, turn right, and continue to the trailhead.

To reach the Mabel trailhead from Clermont, take Route 50 west. The trailhead is at the intersection of Route 50 and CR 772, on the left about five miles west of the Route 50/Bay Lake Road intersection in Mascotte.

Contact: General James A. Van Fleet State Trail
7305 US Highway 27
Clermont, FL 34711
(352) 394-2280
www.dep.state.fl.us/gwt

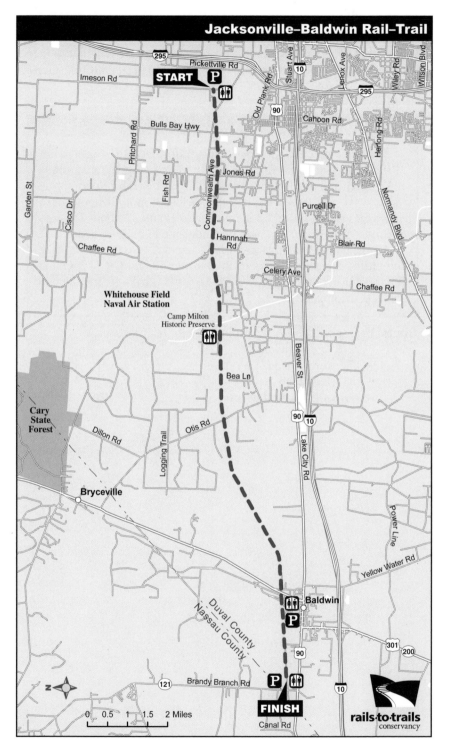

Jacksonville–Baldwin Rail–Trail

START

Imeson Rd
Pickettville Rd
Bulls Bay Hwy
Pritchard Rd
Fish Rd
Jones Rd
Garden St
Cisco Dr
Chaffee Rd
Commonwealth Ave
Hannnah Rd

Old Plank Rd
Stuart Ave
Lenox Ave
Herlong Rd
Wilson Blvd
Wiley Rd

Cahoon Rd
Purcell Dr
Blair Rd
Celery Ave
Chaffee Rd
Normandy Blvd

Whitehouse Field Naval Air Station
Camp Milton Historic Preserve

Bea Ln

Beaver St

Cary State Forest
Dillon Rd
Logging Trail
Otis Rd
Lake City Rd

Bryceville

Power Line
Yellow Water Rd

Duval County
Nassau County

Baldwin

Brandy Branch Rd
FINISH
Canal Rd

rails·to·trails
conservancy

N

0   0.5   1   1.5   2 Miles

Jacksonville–Baldwin Rail-Trail

Just west of bustling downtown Jacksonville, the Jacksonville–Baldwin Rail-Trail, one of north Florida's oldest, traverses a rural setting of hardwood uplands, wetlands, and pine flatwoods. A dense tree canopy shelters much of the nearly 15-mile paved path, providing habitat for hawks, wood storks, stilts, and belted kingfishers. You're also likely to encounter turkeys, alligators, rabbits, gopher tortoises, and coral snakes. Beware of the latter, a venomous species with wide black and red bands broken by narrow yellow rings.

The Imeson Road trailhead, closest to Jacksonville, is a good place to start an out-and-back journey. Here you'll find the first of several restroom facilities and benches along the trail. This spot also marks the start of a separate equestrian trail that runs in the adjacent tree line, except where creek crossings bring trail users together.

Midway along the trail is the Camp Milton Historic Preserve rest area. Once home to the largest encampment of Confederate troops during the Civil War, the site includes the remains of a mile-long defensive works, a re-creation of a late 19th-century homestead, a replica bridge, an arboretum, and extensive boardwalks. Just

Endpoints
Imeson Road to Brandy Branch Road, Jacksonville

Mileage
14.5

Roughness Index
1

Surface
Asphalt

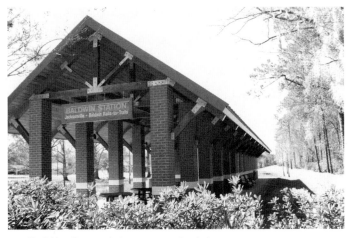

The Baldwin Station trailside rest area provides shade.

west of Camp Milton, you may hear naval aircraft on training runs at nearby Whitehouse Field.

You'll find plenty of restaurants, convenience stores, and gas stations near the trail's eastern endpoint in Jacksonville and at its terminus in Baldwin. Plans are in the works to connect this trail to neighboring recreational and ecological corridors.

DIRECTIONS FROM DOWNTOWN JACKSONVILLE

To reach the Imeson Road trailhead, take I-10 west to Exit 356/I-295 North and head up I-295 to Exit 9/Commonwealth Avenue. Drive west on Commonwealth about a mile to Imeson and turn right. The marked trailhead is on the left.

To reach the Brandy Branch Road trailhead, take I-10 west to Exit 343/US Highway 301 and head north to US Highway 90. Turn left, drive west about two miles, and then turn right on Route 121/Brandy Branch Road. The marked trailhead is on the right.

Contact: City of Jacksonville
Department of Parks, Recreation,
Entertainment, & Conservation
555 West 44th Street
Jacksonville, FL 32208
(904) 630-5400
www.coj.net/Departments/Parks+and+Recreation/
Recreation+Activities/Specialty+Parks/Jacksonville+
Baldwin+Rail+Trail.htm

Nature Coast State Trail

One of the Sunshine State's best-kept trail secrets, the Nature Coast State Trail (formerly the Nature Coast Greenway) connects five small rural towns—Cross City, Old Town, Fanning Springs, Trenton, and Chiefland—along a Y-shaped, 32-mile corridor. From the hub in Fanning Springs, you can take your pick of trips. The well-maintained asphalt path provides enough trailheads, pavilions, and services to ease journeys of any length.

On the 12-mile leg northwest to Cross City via Old Town, pause at viewing areas along the old railroad trestle spanning the Suwannee River. During cooler months, you may spot manatees in the river below.

The seven-mile section of lightly traveled trail east of Fanning Springs leads to the quaint town of Trenton, where you'll find a trailhead, restrooms, nearby businesses, and a colorful railroad mural.

On the nine-mile route southeast to Chiefland, the trail skirts hardwood hammocks along the northern boundary of Andrews Wildlife Management Area. While a few lucky trail users have spotted bobcats, gopher tortoises are a much more common sight.

Endpoints
Cross City, Trenton, and Chiefland

Mileage
32

Roughness Index
1

Surface
Asphalt

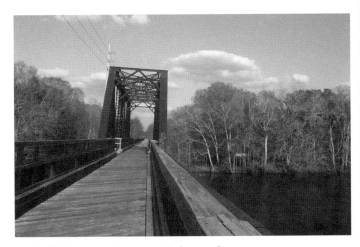

An old railroad trestle takes you over the Suwannee River.

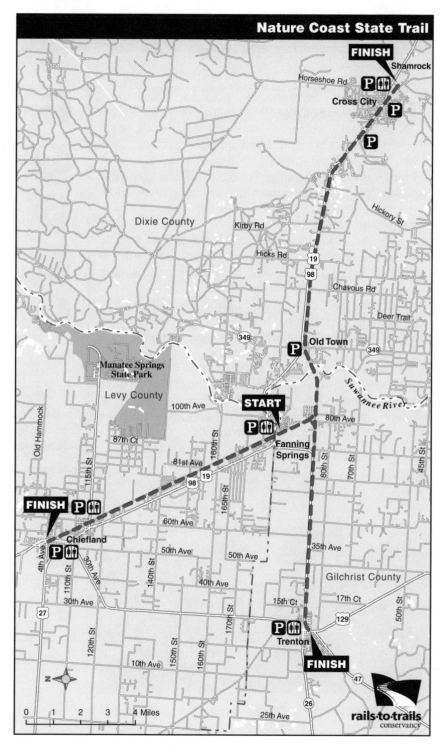

Nature Coast State Trail

FINISH
Shamrock

Horseshoe Rd

Cross City

Dixie County

Kirby Rd

Hicks Rd

19
98

Chavous Rd

Deer Trail

Hickory St

349

Old Town

349

Suwannee River

Manatee Springs
State Park

Levy County

100th Ave

START

80th Ave

Fanning
Springs

87th Ct

81st Ave

19
98

Old Hammock

115th St

160th St

165th St

80th St

70th St

45th St

FINISH

Chiefland

4th Ave

110th St

30th Ave

60th Ave

50th St

50th Ave

140th St

40th Ave

30th Ave

120th St

10th Ave

150th St

160th St

170th St

35th Ave

15th Ct

17th Ct

Gilchrist County

27

129

Trenton

FINISH

47

N

0   1   2   3   4 Miles

25th Ave

26

rails·to·trails
conservancy

Equestrians can access the trail at either the Old Town or Fanning Springs trailheads, where trailer parking is provided. The Fanning Springs trailhead also links up with Fanning Springs State Park, which rewards the weary with refreshing dips in cool spring waters.

Officials are mulling whether to extend the trail south to connect with the Cross-Florida Greenway and the Withlacoochee State Trail (see page 89). Another possibility is an extension east from Trenton to Newberry and, ultimately, Gainesville to connect with other rail-trails.

DIRECTIONS

To reach the Fanning Springs trailhead from Gainesville, take Route 26 west about 40 miles to Fanning Springs. At the T-junction with US Highway 19/98, turn right. The trailhead lies just east of the Suwannee River.

To reach the Cross City trailhead from Fanning Springs, take US Highway 19/98 north about 13 miles to Cross City, then turn east on Route 351, the last intersection before the old train depot. The trail crosses this road.

To reach the Old Town trailhead from Fanning Springs, take US Highway 19/98 four miles west to Old Town and turn north on Route 349. The trailhead is one block up, adjacent to the fire station.

To reach the Trenton trailhead from Fanning Springs, take Route 26 eight miles east to Trenton and turn north on US Highway 129. The trailhead is two blocks up at the old train depot.

To reach the Chiefland trailhead, take US Highway 19/98 south to Chiefland. The trailhead is at the old train depot, two blocks south of downtown on the same road.

Contact: Office of Greenways & Trails
18020 NW Highway 19
Fanning Springs, FL 32693
(352) 493-6072
www.dep.state.fl.us/gwt/guide/regions/crossflorida/
trails/nature_coast_trail%20.htm

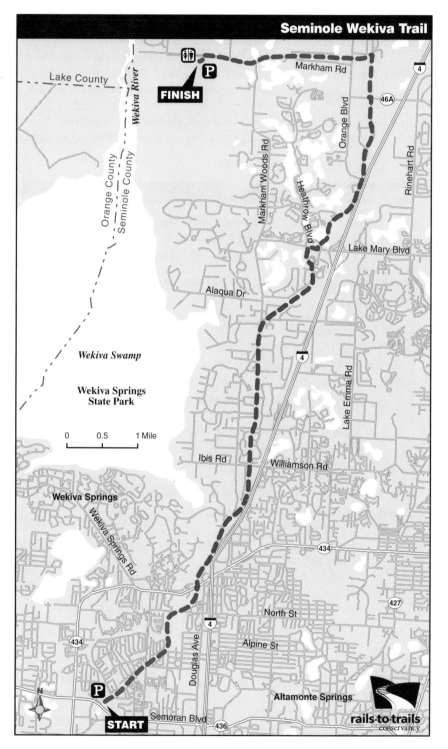

Seminole Wekiva Trail

Markham Rd

Lake County

Wekiva River

4

46A

Orange Blvd

Rinehart Rd

Markham Woods Rd

Heathrow Blvd

FINISH

Orange County
Seminole County

Lake Mary Blvd

Alaqua Dr

Wekiva Swamp

**Wekiva Springs
State Park**

0   0.5   1 Mile

Lake Emma Rd

Ibis Rd

Williamson Rd

4

Wekiva Springs

Wekiva Springs Rd

434

434

North St

427

I-4

Alpine St

Douglas Ave

P

START

Semoran Blvd

436

Altamonte Springs

rails·to·trails
conservancy

Seminole Wekiva Trail

Running along the former line of the Orange Belt Railway, the Seminole Wekiva Trail offers a peaceful alternative to the busy streets of Altamonte Springs. This popular, well-marked 14-mile route is one of Seminole County's showcase trails.

From Altamonte Springs, the trail begins across a pleasant wooden bridge at the San Sebastian Prado trailhead. The first seven miles traverse quiet residential neighborhoods and lush woods. Draped with Spanish moss, the tree canopy provides welcome shade. Two miles in you'll reach the ball fields and open park space of the Seminole County Softball Complex.

North of Mile Marker 7 the mood shifts from rural relaxation to suburban bustle. Over the next three miles, you'll skirt the International Parkway business corridor, weaving amid modern office buildings and shopping centers with ample food, water, and restroom options. Just past Mile Marker 9, a spur trail on the right leads east to a pedestrian bridge over I-4 before joining the Cross-Seminole Trail (see page 41).

The final four miles of the Seminole Wekiva mirror the peaceful wooded areas that began the trail. At trail's end, the Markham Road trailhead offers ample parking and restroom facilities.

Endpoints
Altamonte Springs to Wekiva River Protection Area (west of Sanford)

Mileage
14

Roughness Index
1

Surface
Asphalt

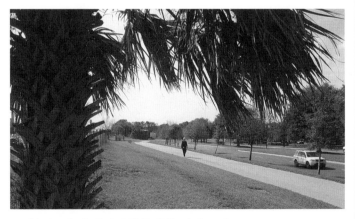

Palm trees line the Seminole Wekiva Trail's suburban path.

DIRECTIONS

To reach the San Sebastian Prado trailhead, take I-4 to Exit 92 and drive west about 1.5 miles on Route 436/Semoran Boulevard. The well-marked trailhead is on the north side of the boulevard.

To reach the Markham Road trailhead, take I-4 to Exit 101 and head west on Route 46A. Turn right on Orange Boulevard, then left on Markham. The marked trailhead is on the left.

Parking is available at both trailheads.

Contact: Seminole County Trails & Greenways
520 West Lake Mary Blvd., Suite 200
Sanford, FL 32773
(407) 665-2093
www.seminolecountyfl.gov/pw/trails/
trails_semwekiva.asp

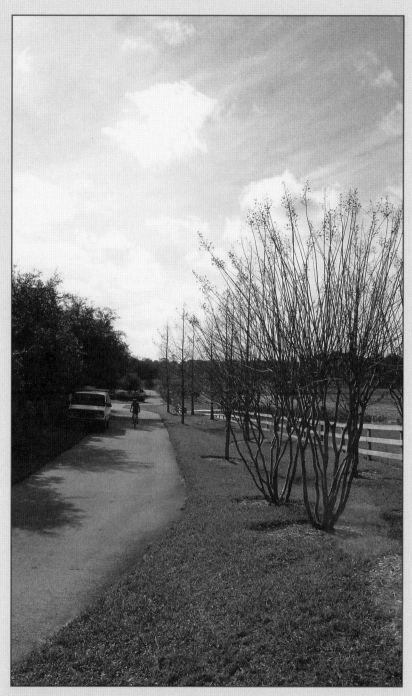

Flowering trees bloom on the wide Seminole Wekiva Trail.

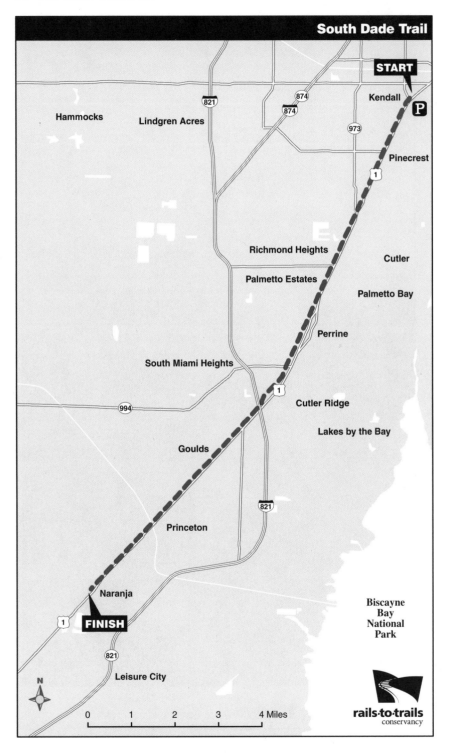

South Dade Trail

START

Kendall

P

Hammocks

Lindgren Acres

821

874

874

973

Pinecrest

1

Richmond Heights

Cutler

Palmetto Estates

Palmetto Bay

Perrine

South Miami Heights

994

1

Cutler Ridge

Lakes by the Bay

Goulds

821

Princeton

Naranja

1

FINISH

Biscayne
Bay
National
Park

Leisure City

821

N

0   1   2   3   4 Miles

rails·to·trails
conservancy

South Dade Trail

component of the commuter corridor between Miami and South Dade County, this trail is nothing short of an urban adventure. Paralleling US Highway 1 for most of its length, the 13.5-mile route was adapted for—and is largely used by—urban commuters seeking refuge from Miami's heavy traffic congestion. The trail connects such points of interest as the Dadeland and Cutler Ridge shopping areas and commercial office spaces. It also links up with the Metrobus and Metrorail lines.

Cyclists can stretch their legs on this fairly open trail, but you must wait your turn and use caution when crossing its many major intersections. Metrobus stations along the route provide plenty of parking, so you can pick up the trail just about anywhere. Dadeland Mall anchors the north end, Cutler Mall is about 8.5 miles south, and the trail ends another five miles south at SW 264th Street.

The trail is slated to extend another five miles south along the bus route to Homestead. From there, it will eventually reach Florida City along a section of Henry Flagler's famed Florida East Coast Railway, which once

Endpoints
Dadeland Mall to
SW 264th Street

Mileage
13.5

Roughness Index
1

Surface
Asphalt

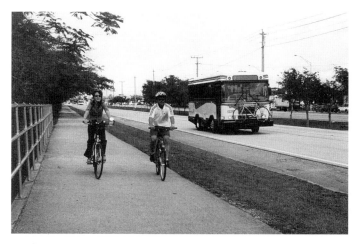

Commuting by bike is a breeze on the South Dade Trail.

67

stretched from Jacksonville to Key West. Another planned extension to the north will connect with the M-Path rail-with-trail.

Big future plans aside, the best aspect of this trail is that all Miami-Dade Metrobuses provide bicycle racks, for which they do not require special permits. So, after a long day of riding, walking, shopping, or sitting at your desk, simply mount your bike on the rack at the front of the bus, pay your fare, and climb aboard—you've earned the air-conditioned return trip.

DIRECTIONS

Dadeland Mall is on US Highway 1, just south of downtown Miami. The trail parallels the highway to the west.

The trailhead at SW 264th Street is on the west side of the highway, midway between Miami and Homestead.

Contact: Miami-Dade Metropolitan Planning Organization
111 NW First Street, Suite 910
Miami, FL 33128
(305) 375-4507
www.miamidade.gov/mpo/home.htm

South Lake Trail

About 20 miles west of Orlando, the South Lake Trail (a.k.a. Lake Minneola Scenic Trail) takes in some of central Florida's most spectacular prospects. Nowhere in this region will you find more hills, lakes, and wide-open vistas than along this seven-mile paved trail. As an added bonus, the trail is only five miles from the West Orange Trail, and plans are afoot to connect the two. At the trail midpoint, signs point to a quarter mile spur for the Minneola trailhead, a good spot to park your car.

The trail starts atop a hill near Lake-Sumter Community College on North Hancock Road. On a clear day you'll have wonderful views of the entire region, from glimmering lakes to the Orlando skyline. The first two miles are an easy downhill toward Lake Minneola in Clermont. Streetlamps allow for safe nighttime use on this heavily used section.

Down on the lake, the trail skirts the south shore, offering beautiful views. Clermont Public Beach boasts cool water and such trailside amenities as restrooms, picnic tables, and parking. The final mile wraps around the lake to the western trailhead. Any of the side streets leading away from the lake will take you to the shops and restaurants of downtown Clermont.

Endpoints
North Hancock
Road to
Clermont

Mileage
7

**Roughness
Index**
1

Surface
Asphalt

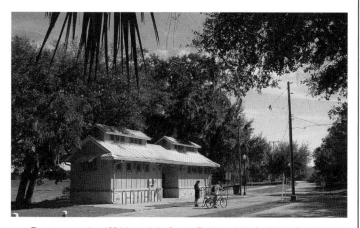

There are more than 100 lakes in Lake County, Florida, and the South Lake Trail skirts the impressive Lake Minneola.

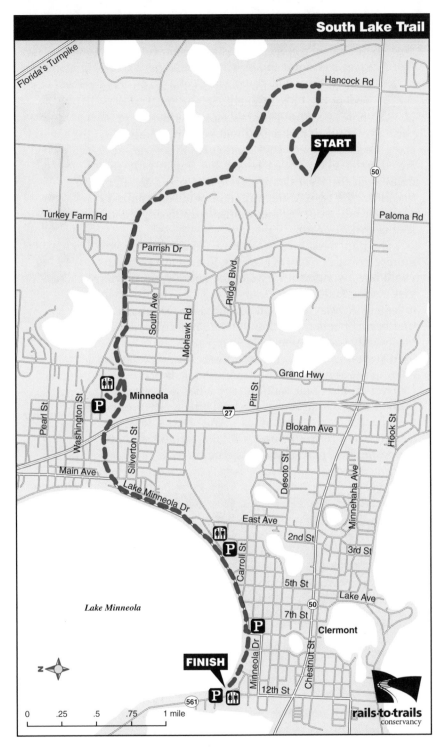

DIRECTIONS

To reach the Minneola trailhead from Route 561 in Clermont, skirt the south shore of the lake, turn right on Washington Street/Old Highway 50, and continue east until you see signs for the trail.

To reach the western trailhead, take Route 50 to 12th Street in Clermont and head north half a mile. The trailhead entrance is on the right.

Parking is available at both trailheads.

Contact: City of Minneola
P.O. Box 678
Minneola, FL 34755
(352) 394-3898

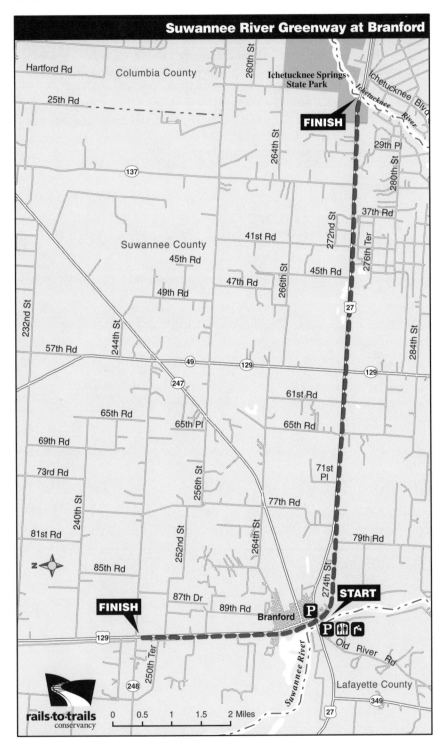

Suwannee River Greenway at Branford

Hartford Rd

Columbia County

25th Rd

137

Suwannee County

45th Rd

49th Rd

232nd St

57th Rd

244th St

49

247

65th Rd

69th Rd

73rd Rd

240th St

81st Rd

85th Rd

87th Dr

FINISH

129

248

Ichetucknee Springs
State Park

Ichetucknee Blvd

Ichetucknee River

FINISH

260th St

264th St

29th Pl

280th St

37th Rd

41st Rd

272nd St

276th Ter

45th Rd

47th Rd

266th St

45th Rd

27

284th St

129

129

61st Rd

65th Pl

65th Rd

256th St

71st
Pl

77th Rd

264th St

79th Rd

252nd St

274th St

START

89th Rd

Branford

P

P

Old River Rd

Lafayette County

349

Suwannee River

27

250th Ter

rails·to·trails
conservancy

0   0.5   1   1.5   2 Miles

Suwannee River Greenway at Branford

Following a former CSX Railroad corridor, this 11.5-mile paved trail runs from just east of the Suwannee River to the west bank of the Ichetucknee River. Along the way, numerous benches and small covered pavilions beneath a dense tree canopy provide plenty of shady rest stops.

Both trailheads—at Ivey Memorial Park and in Branford—lie in a bend along the western half of the trail. Ivey holds the only public restroom and water fountain, so you may want to start your trip here. Consider a visit to Branford's restaurants, convenience stores, and gas stations before hitting the trail.

North of town, the trail parallels US Highway 129 for about 2.5 miles before it ends. If you continue west just over a mile along lightly traveled CR 248, you'll reach Little River Springs State Park. Cool off with a dip in the springs at this slice of old Florida on the Suwannee.

Heading back toward Branford along the trail, you'll pass the trailheads before reaching a gopher tortoise preserve at the trail midpoint. Be on the lookout for a gopher tortoise or two, as well as other small trail critters.

Endpoints
US Highway 129
and CR 248 to
Ichetucknee River

Mileage
11.5

**Roughness
Index**
2

Surface
Asphalt

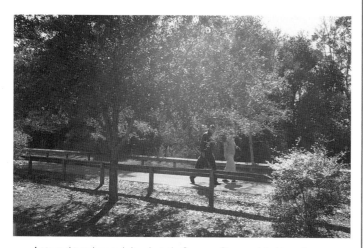

A trip on this trail can include a dip in the Suwannee River or a tube trip on the Ichetucknee River.

The eastern half is a bit rough, particularly where it parallels the road and rails; there's less debris on the portions built directly atop the abandoned line.

By the time you reach the trail's end, you may be ready for a relaxing tube ride down the meandering Ichetucknee River. Also worth a visit is Ichetucknee Springs State Park, a short drive away.

DIRECTIONS

To reach the Branford trailhead, take US Highway 27 north to US Highway 129, turn north, then take the first left on Trail Street/Owens Avenue. Parking is at road's end.

Ivey Memorial Park is on the other side of US Highway 27, just east of the Suwannee River.

Contact: Suwannee County Recreation Department
1201 Silas Drive
Live Oak, FL 32064
(386) 362-3004
www.suwanneeparksandrecreation.org

Tallahassee–St. Marks Historic Railroad State Trail

The first rail-trail developed by the state, Tallahassee–St. Marks Historic Railroad State Trail follows the route of Florida's first and longest-operating railroad, used primarily to transport cotton from plantations to waiting ships. Today, adventure awaits along the trail and in nearby state parks.

As its name implies, the trail stretches from the capital city south to coastal St. Marks. Longleaf pine and forests of oak, wax myrtle, and yaupon holly offer attractive, welcome shade.

From the Capital Circle trailhead, the path leads 4.5 miles north to within blocks of Florida State University and the two-mile Stadium Drive Bike Path, a favorite among students. While this section offers few facilities, plenty of services line the route.

The first few miles south of the trailhead can get somewhat congested, particularly on weekends. Just remember proper trail etiquette and have a good time. If you're riding a mountain bike, consider a spin at the Munson Hills Off-Road Trail, about a mile from the trailhead (mileage is painted on the asphalt). While this loop

Endpoints
Tallahassee
to St. Marks

Mileage
20

Roughness Index
1

Surface
Asphalt

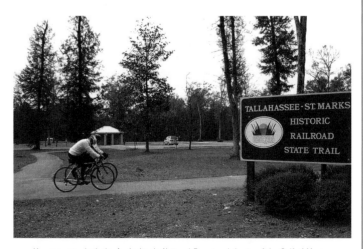

You can enjoy both the Apalachicola National Forest and the tip of the Gulf of Mexico on this trail.

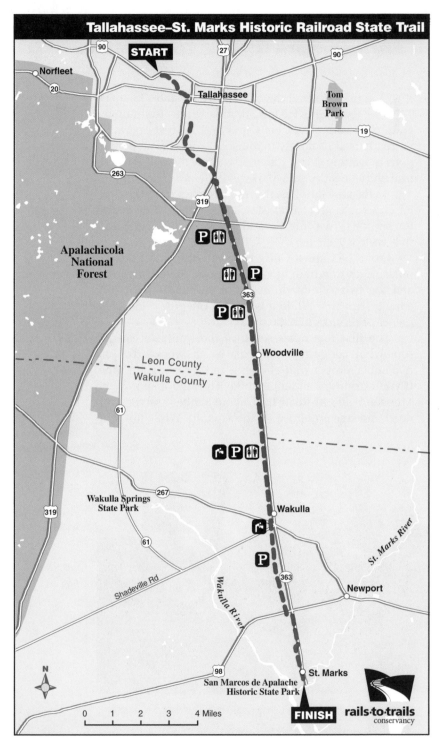

Tallahassee–St. Marks Historic Railroad State Trail

can get a bit sandy during dry months, the scenery and remote terrain make it worthwhile.

Near Mile Marker 9, Wakulla Station trailhead provides water, shelter, and restrooms. A bit farther south, a five-mile detour along the paved shoulder of Route 267 leads to Wakulla Springs State Park, known for its big, beautiful spring and refreshing swimming hole.

About six miles farther down the trail, you'll emerge in St. Marks. Consider continuing south and west of trail's end to visit San Marcos de Apalache Historic State Park. Otherwise, simply hit one of the waterfront restaurants to wet your whistle and carb-load with friends while watching boats ply the St. Marks River.

DIRECTIONS

The Capital Circle trailhead is on the west side of Route 363/Woodville Highway in Tallahassee, just south of Capital Circle.

Trail access and parking is also available at Woodville Sports Complex on the west side of the trail off Route 363/Woodville Highway. Follow the brown directional signs south to the complex.

The Wakulla Station trailhead is on the west side of the trail off Route 363/Woodville Highway, just south of the Leon/Wakulla county line. Follow the brown directional signs south to the trailhead.

Contact: Tallahassee–St. Marks Historic Railroad State Trail
3900 Commonwealth Blvd., MS 795
Tallahassee, FL 32399
(850) 245-2052
www.dep.state.fl.us/gwt/guide/regions/
panhandleeast/trails/tallahassee_stmarks.htm

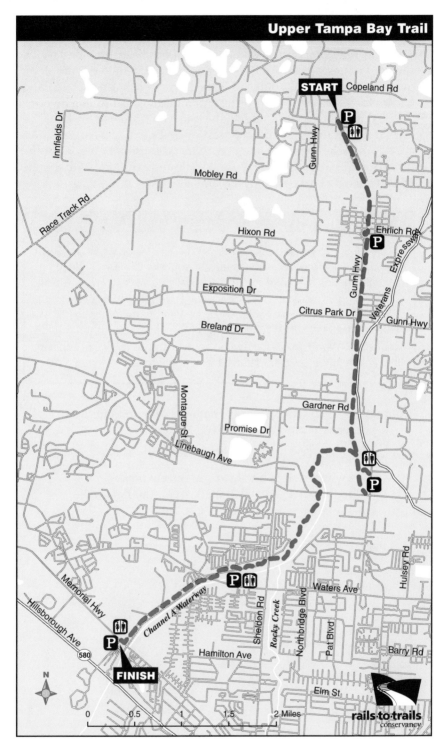

Upper Tampa Bay Trail

Widely regarded as Tampa Bay's best urban trail, the Upper Tampa Bay Trail (a.k.a. Suncoast Trail) provides a scenic escape from its congested surroundings. The original section winds through suburban Citrus Park on an unused railroad corridor and extends along the west bank of the Channel A waterway, a newly constructed drainage canal.

From the Peterson Park trailhead, the first mile leads through a rural landscape past grazing cattle, sheep, and other livestock. At Ehrlich Road the scene waxes suburban, and interesting local eateries tempt you with their fare. Next, you're transported over busy Gunn Highway on a beautifully constructed pedestrian bridge, a good example of Florida's investment in its local trails.

The route then diverts from the original railroad corridor and takes a sharp right onto the recently opened section along the Channel A waterway, lined with native vegetation and beautiful cypress trees. You'll soon cross a lovely wooden bridge over peaceful Rocky Creek.

Continue following the west bank to the Waters Avenue trailhead, which offers plenty of parking, restroom facilities, and an information center. This is a good spot

Endpoints
Peterson Park
Road to Memorial
Highway

Mileage
8

Roughness Index
1

Surface
Asphalt

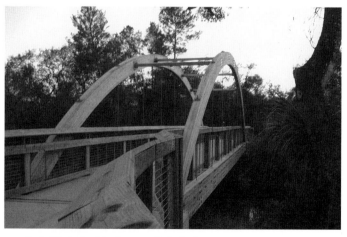

A refurbished railroad trestle crosses Rocky Creek.

to begin a trek or take a break. Beyond, the trail crosses Waters Avenue and parallels Memorial Highway to the westernmost trailhead.

DIRECTIONS FROM DOWNTOWN TAMPA

To reach the Peterson Park trailhead, take Veterans Expressway north to Exit 10/Ehrlich Road, head west a mile and turn right on Gunn Highway. Drive a mile north on Gunn Highway and turn right on Peterson Road. The trailhead is in the park.

To reach the Memorial Highway trailhead, take Veterans Expressway north to Exit 4/Hillsborough Avenue West/Route 580. Drive west five miles and turn right on Countryway Boulevard. After a half mile, turn right on Memorial Highway. The trailhead is on the left.

Contact: Hillsborough County Parks
Recreation & Conservation Department
101 East River Cove Street
Tampa, FL 33604
(813) 275-7275
www.hillsboroughcounty.org/parks

Waldo Road Greenway, Depot Avenue Rail-Trail, & Kermit Sigmon Bike Trail

The Waldo Road Greenway, Depot Avenue Rail-Trail, and Kermit Sigmon Bike Trail have been seamlessly connected as part of Gainesville's ever-expanding rail-trail network. Together, the three comprise a 6.7-mile network that links neighborhoods, businesses, transit stops, a private aviation terminal, and the University of Florida campus. They'll soon connect with the scenic Gainesville–Hawthorne State Trail (see p. 47). While there are no formal trailheads or parking areas, you can access the route from a number of road crossings. (The Gainesville Depot is being restored to serve as a formal trailhead.)

Starting from the north at Waldo Road and NE 47th Avenue, the Waldo Road Greenway is particularly well landscaped and passes numerous public transportation connections. Be aware that the trail narrows at intersections and at a couple of the transit stops.

The Depot Avenue Rail-Trail picks up just over two miles from the Waldo Road/University Avenue intersection. Threading through neighborhoods and industrial areas, it never loses its community essence. Be sure to check out the colorful murals on the 13th Street trestle, a relic from the rail line that once crossed

Endpoints
Within Gainesville

Mileage
6.7

Roughness Index
1

Surface
Asphalt

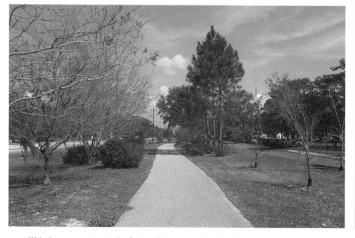

With three connecting trails, Gainesville is a growing rail-trail town.

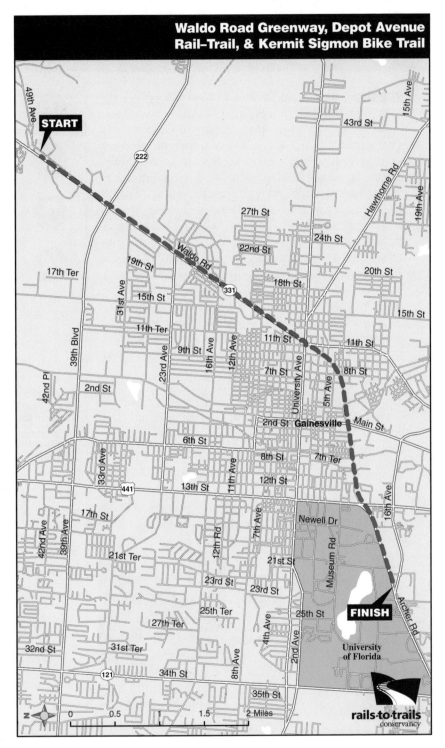

Waldo Road Greenway, Depot Avenue Rail–Trail, & Kermit Sigmon Bike Trail

START

FINISH

Gainesville

University of Florida

rails·to·trails
conservancy

the state from Fernandina Beach on the Atlantic Ocean to Cedar Key on the Gulf of Mexico.

Across the trestle, you'll join the Kermit Sigmon Bike Trail. Named for a local doctor, the trail leads west past both Shands and Veterans hospitals, and hospital employees use it as a commuter corridor. Although the route continues another two miles west, it's probably best to end your trip here; the Archer Road crossing poses a significant hazard, and its narrow sidewalk flanks the wrong side of the road for westbound cyclists.

DIRECTIONS

The route offers numerous access points, particularly along Waldo and Archer roads, where the trail intersects with SW 13th and South Main streets, and on several side streets.

Contact: City of Gainesville
Public Works Department
P.O. Box 490, MS 58
Gainesville, FL 32602
(352) 334-5074
www.cityofgainesville.org/pubworks

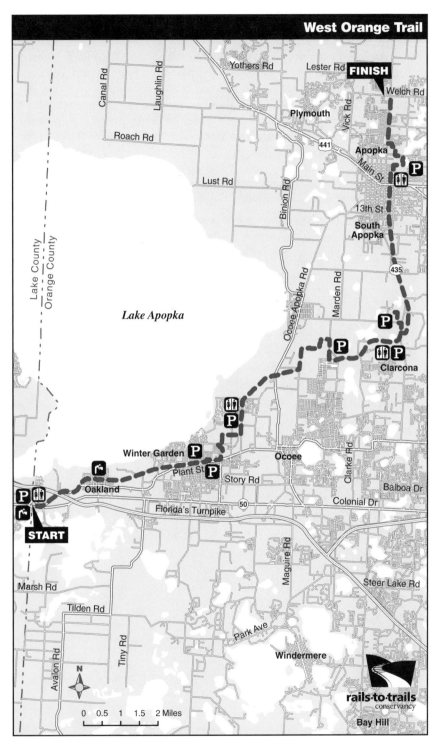

West Orange Trail

Connecting small communities and suburban neighborhoods, the 22-mile West Orange Trail is one of Florida's most popular rail-trails, thanks to its reputation and proximity to metro Orlando. Fifteen minutes northwest of downtown, the route serves as a window on the region's past and present, passing through 1950s communities that grew up around the once-thriving Orange Belt Railway, as well as more developed areas in this rapidly expanding metropolitan area.

Killarney Station, a modern take on an old-time train depot, anchors the southern trailhead. Here you'll find bike rentals, restrooms, and water. From here the route leads northeast through the quiet, wooded community of Oakland before hitting downtown Winter Garden. For about a mile the trail threads down the middle of two-lane Plant Street, allowing trail users to browse the shops and restaurants of this lively community.

Over the next 10 miles the trail pops in and out of thinly wooded areas, occasionally passing orange groves that speak to the county's agricultural roots. This stretch is open to equestrian use.

Endpoints
Orange/Lake county line to Welch Road

Mileage
22

Roughness Index
1

Surface
Concrete, asphalt, woodchips, dirt

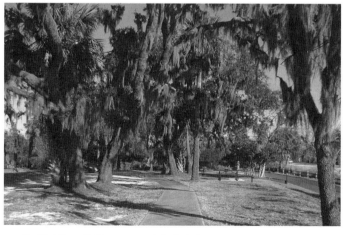

The West Orange Trail has won awards for its design.

Beyond lies Apopka, one of central Florida's fastest growing communities. You'll soon cross busy US Highway 441 along Forest Avenue. Use caution here until the planned pedestrian bridge is in place. The trail runs three more miles along North Park Avenue before ending at the northern trailhead on East Welch Road.

DIRECTIONS FROM ORLANDO

To reach the Killarney Station trailhead, take Florida's Turnpike to Exit 272, and head west on Route 50/West Colonial Drive. In less than a mile, turn right on Deer Island Road and take the next left on Old SR 50 East. Killarney Station is a half-mile ahead on the left. Parking is available.

To reach the northern trailhead, take I-4 to Route 50/West Colonial Drive and head west. Within a mile, turn right on US Highway 441 and drive north 11.5 miles to Route 435. Turn right on Route 435 and look for the trailhead 2.25 miles ahead on the right, where Route 435 and East Welch Road intersect. While there is no parking at this trailhead, you can park along the route.

Contact: West Orange Trail–Chapin Station
501 Crown Point Cross Road
Winter Garden, FL 34787
(407) 654-1108
www.orangecountyfl.net/dept/cesrvcs/
parks/parkdetails.asp?parkid=44

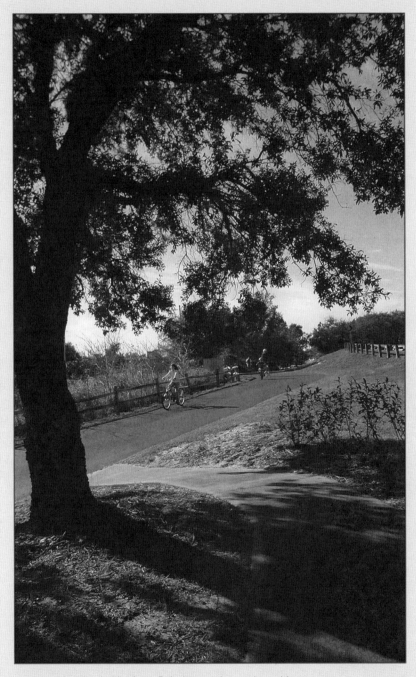

Its gentle grade makes the West Orange Trail a fun, easy place to ride your bike.

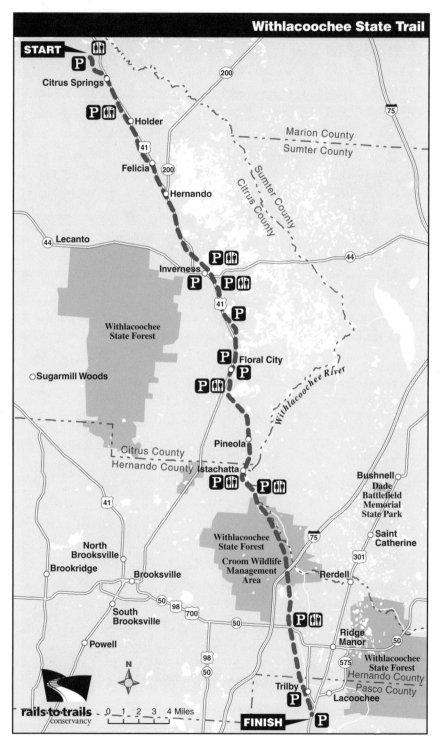

Withlacoochee State Trail

Withlacoochee State Trail

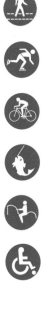

Forty-six-mile Withlacoochee State Trail is a must-do, pure Florida experience for any trail enthusiast. Situated between Orlando and Tampa, it hosts a steady stream of visitors and locals on its paved path and adjacent equestrian trail.

The Withlacoochee's length, popularity, and proximity to numerous communities have given rise to seven trailheads, information kiosks, colorful murals, and convenient parks. Although the trail makes for a long journey, food and drink are never too far as you travel southbound through Citrus Springs, Inverness, Floral City, Istachatta, and Trilby.

For much of its length, the trail parallels the Withlacoochee River, a state-designated paddling trail. The best place to catch river views and put in your canoe or kayak is at Nobelton Wayside Park, about eight miles south of Floral City. From here the trail crosses the Withlacoochee State Forest and Croom Wildlife Management Area. In the mornings and early evenings expect to see deer along this roughly six-mile stretch. Near the southern boundary, Silver Lake Recreation Area offers year-round camping.

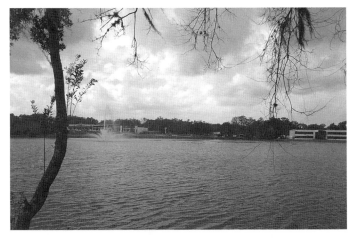

Currently, the Withlacoochee State Trail is Florida's longest rail-trail.

Endpoints
Gulf Junction to Owensboro Junction

Mileage
46

Roughness Index
1

Surface
Asphalt

Several miles farther south is the heavily trafficked Ridge Manor trailhead, just off US Highway 98/Route 50. Fortunately, a state-of-the-art overpass leads safely across the congested roadway. There are no further road crossings over the final six miles to Trilby and the Owensboro Junction trailhead.

DIRECTIONS

To reach the Gulf Junction trailhead from Dunnellon, take US Highway 41 south and turn right on Magenta Drive. Follow Magenta to the marked trailhead on the left.

To reach the South Citrus Springs trailhead, continue south on US Highway 41 to South Citrus Springs Boulevard and head west one block. The trailhead is on the left.

To reach the Inverness trailhead, continue south on US Highway 41 to Inverness and turn left on North Apopka Avenue. The marked trailhead is a few blocks up North Apopka.

To reach the Ridge Manor trailhead, take I-75 to Exit 61 and head east on US Highway 98/Route 50. After about a mile, turn left on Croom Rital Road and look for the trailhead on the right.

To reach the Trilby trailhead, continue east on Route 50 to Route 575/Burwell Road and turn right. The trailhead is a half mile farther, where the road and trail intersect.

To reach the Owensboro Junction trailhead from Trilby, head south on US Highway 301/98. The trailhead lies just south of town on the right.

Contact: Withlacoochee State Trail
315 North Apopka Avenue
Inverness, FL 34450
(352) 726-2251
www.dep.state.fl.us/gwt/state/with/default.htm

You can easily make a vacation out of a trip on the Withlacoochee State Trail with its lush parks, trailside eateries, and historical railroad relics, as well as the cool waters of the nearby Withlacoochee River.

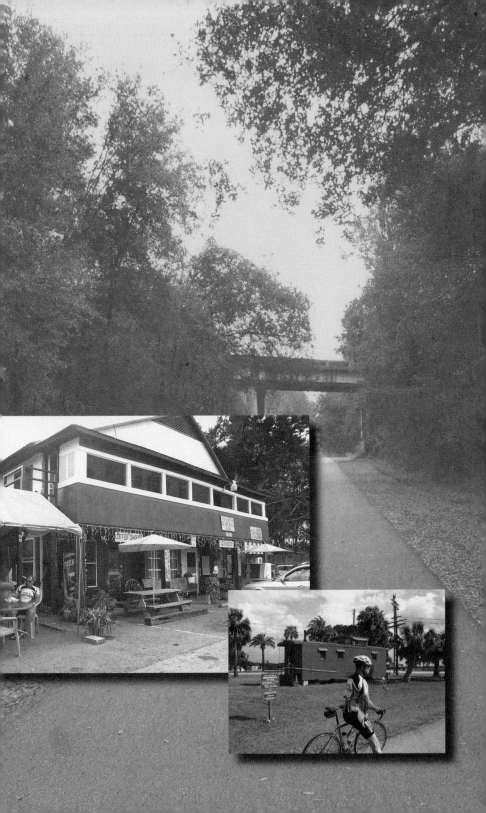

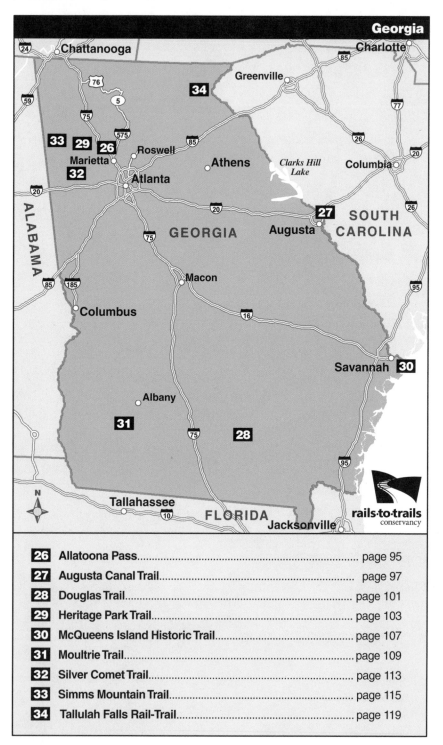

Georgia

Georgia

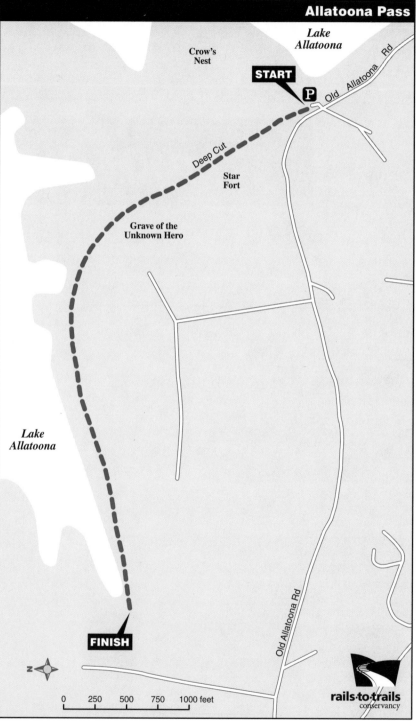

Allatoona Pass

Lake
Allatoona

Crow's
Nest

START

P

Old Allatoona Rd

Deep Cut

Star
Fort

Grave of the
Unknown Hero

Lake
Allatoona

FINISH

Old Allatoona Rd

N

0   250   500   750   1000 feet

rails·to·trails
conservancy

Allatoona Pass

While mile-long Allatoona Pass is today a serene, pine-shaded trail, in April 1862 it played a role in the Great Locomotive Chase, when disguised Union soldiers seeking to destroy critical bridges along the Western & Atlantic line tore through in *The General*, a stolen Confederate locomotive. The pass also witnessed a bloody Civil War battle and holds the Grave of the Unknown Hero, burial site of an unidentified Confederate soldier. The packed dirt surface and multitude of historical markers make this a fascinating place for a leisurely day hike.

Within minutes of starting your hike, you'll enter the shady reaches of Deep Cut, a 95-foot-long man-made gorge, its rock walls looming 170 feet overhead. Beyond it you'll encounter the first of several side trails, a set of stairs on the left that climb to Star Fort. Highlights include markers that detail the Battle of Allatoona Pass and an antique photograph of the view Union soldiers had from this very spot.

Several yards up the main trail, a side path on the right leads to a lookout station known as the Crow's Nest, where a massive tree visible from Kennesaw

Endpoints
Allatoona Pass, Cartersville

Mileage
1

Roughness Index
2

Surface
Dirt

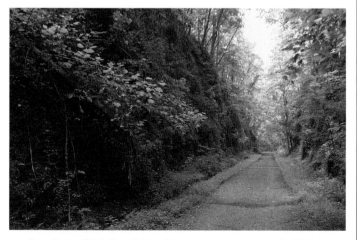

Enter Allatoona Pass's "Deep Cut"—made for the trains to pass through the hillside.

Mountain served as a signal tower. Farther along, a short path on the right leads to vast Lake Allatoona, hemmed in by mountains. Trail's end is marked by a gate, which you can bypass to stroll the scenic lakeshore.

DIRECTIONS

Take I-75 to Exit 283 and head east on Old Allatoona Road for 1.5 miles. Cross the railroad tracks and continue another mile to markers for Allatoona Pass Battlefield on the left. Parking is available here.

Contact: Etowah Valley Historical Society
P.O. Box 1886
Cartersville, GA 30120
(770) 606-8862
www.evhsonline.org

Augusta Canal Trail

This 7.5-mile trail occupies a unique historic and natural setting in the heart of Augusta. Originally constructed in 1845, the waterway itself is the only unbroken, still accessible industrial canal in the South. Its textile heritage is preserved in several existing period structures, including ornate Sibley Mill and a Confederate-era parapet. The trail is part of the larger Augusta Canal National Heritage Area, featuring the Augusta Canal Interpretive Center.

The packed-dirt trail runs along a strip of green between the canal and the Savannah River, where small rapids cascade over granite ledges separating the coastal plain from the Piedmont plateau. Starting from the outskirts of downtown, the trail passes Sibley Mill, enters a lightly developed neighborhood, and then really turns on the charm along a tree-canopied segment beyond an I-20 underpass. You would never know you're just a stone's throw from downtown Augusta. The shady forest and adjacent cool waterways offer relief in the steamy summer months.

Trailside activities include boat tours of the Savannah River, canoe rentals, and mountain biking on trails

Endpoints
King and Sibley mills to Augusta Canal National Heritage Center

Mileage
7.5

Roughness Index
2

Surface
Asphalt, dirt, grass

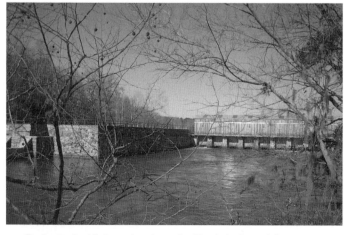

The Augusta Canal Trail runs along the canal and beside the Savannah River.

97

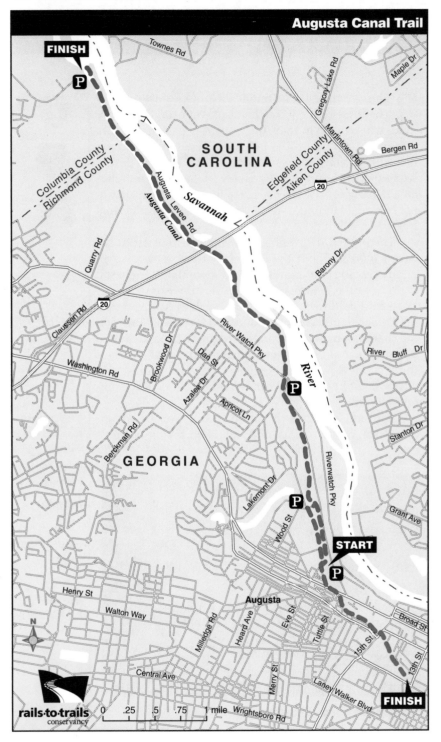

that parallel the main route. Cross over either bridge at the southern parking areas to continue your stroll. The trail ends at the scenic Savannah Rapids Park.

DIRECTIONS

From downtown Augusta, take Broad Street west to Goodrich Street and turn right. Continue just under a mile to a parking lot at the pumping station adjacent to the King and Sibley mills.

Contact: Augusta Canal Authority
P.O. Box 2367
Augusta, GA 30903
(706) 823-0440
(888) 659-8926
www.augustacanal.com

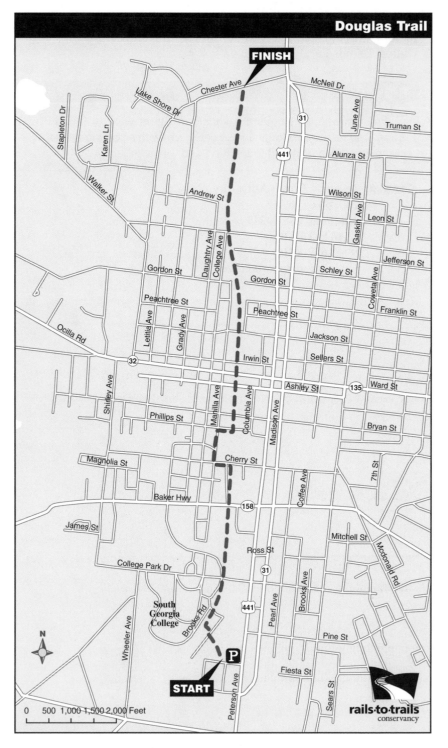

Douglas Trail

About 135 miles southwest of Savannah, rural Douglas has successfully transformed its railroad line, a former economic generator, into a multi-use trail. Built atop the bed of the old Georgia & Florida Railroad, the three-mile trail serves as a transportation corridor and recreational hub for the town's 11,000 residents.

From the West Coffee Middle School trailhead, the route meanders past tennis courts and a baseball field and crosses the landscaped campus of South Georgia College, the state's oldest junior college. Beyond is an eclectic mix of single-family homes, businesses, old farmhouses, mobile homes, and warehouses. While road crossings are plentiful on this trail, they're clearly marked for safe use.

Midway along the trail on Ward Street West you'll pass the old train depot, now the Heritage Station Museum (open Tuesday through Friday as well as every first and third Saturday). Stop in to learn about the railroad that once ran through Douglas and contributed so much to the local economy.

Endpoints
West Coffee Middle
School to North
Chester Avenue

Mileage
3

**Roughness
Index**
1

Surface
Asphalt

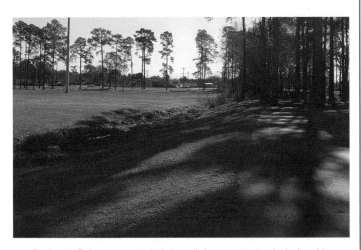

The Douglas Trail is a community trail above all else, connecting local schools and homes.

101

Continuing along a path lined with sweet-smelling pines, you'll soon reach trail's end at North Chester Avenue. Linger on the return trip to appreciate the pleasant landscaping or take a breather on one of the trailside benches.

DIRECTIONS

To reach the West Coffee Middle School trailhead (1303 Peterson Avenue South), take GA 32/Ward Street East and turn left on Peterson. Parking is available.

The Heritage Station Museum (219 Ward Street West) is on the north side of GA 32/Ward Street West, two blocks west of Peterson Avenue. Parking is available.

Contact: City of Douglas
200-C South Madison Avenue
Douglas, GA 31533
(912) 389-3433
www.cityofdouglas.com

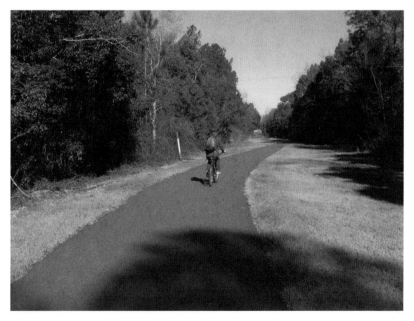

Pine trees lend their sweet smell to a bike ride on the Douglas Trail.

Heritage Park Trail

The Heritage Park Trail links two paths at the confluence of the Oostanaula and Etowah rivers, where these two waterways meet to form the Coosa River. Paved promenades line either side of the Oostanaula, and a railroad trestle overlooking the confluence has been converted into a pedestrian bridge. It forms the bottom curve of this U-shaped trail.

Start your trek by heading down to Unity Point, east of the pedestrian bridge, for views of the layered pathways and gardens and the rivers below. From the west side of the bridge the trail winds about two miles along the Oostanaula. While it ends amid a rather dull residential district, the return trip offers beautiful views of the tree-lined river and historic brick buildings in downtown Rome.

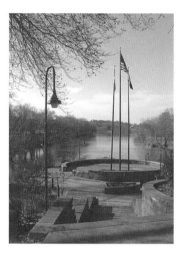

Views of the Oostanaula River dominate the Heritage Park Trail, and you cross at the convergence of the Oostanaula and Coosa rivers.

Sail past your starting point and skirt the east bank of the Oostanaula for even more trailside gems. This route saunters along the river, offering scenic lookouts and several diversions. You'll wander through wooded stretches and pleasant parks and pass baseball fields, volleyball courts, playgrounds, a boat dock, and a fishing area.

Just north of Ridge Ferry Park, a spur trail leads to the Chieftains Museum, a National Historic Landmark that highlights the culture and heritage of the Cherokee Indians. Follow the spur to Riverside Parkway; the museum is on a corner across the street. The onward trail emerges at State Mutual Stadium, where with good timing, you might catch nine innings of the Rome Braves, a minor league affiliate of the Atlanta Braves.

Endpoints
First Avenue and Broad Street to Veterans Memorial Parkway, Rome

Mileage
4.5

Roughness Index
1

Surface
Asphalt

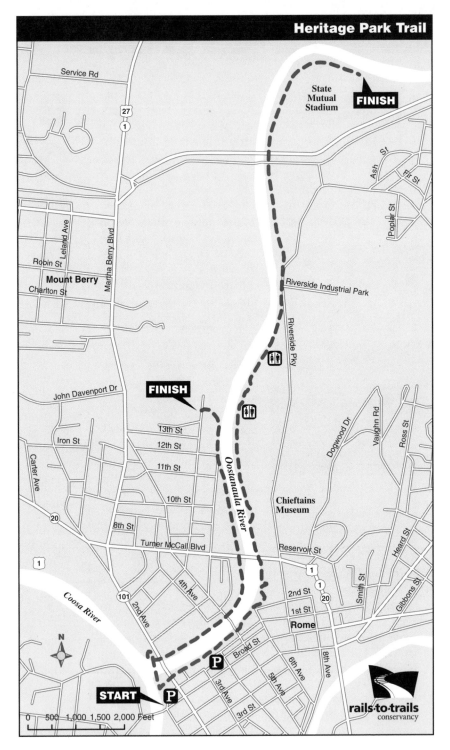

DIRECTIONS

To reach Heritage Park, take GA 20 to Second Avenue, head south, and turn right on Broad Street. You'll find parking one block down on the right.

To reach the State Mutual Stadium trailhead, take I-75 to Exit 200, head west on Highway 411, and turn right on Veterans Memorial Highway. The stadium is at the intersection of Veterans Memorial and Riverside Parkway. Parking is available.

Contact: Rome–Floyd Parks & Recreation Authority
300 West Third Street
Rome, GA 30165
(706) 291-0766
www.rfpra.com

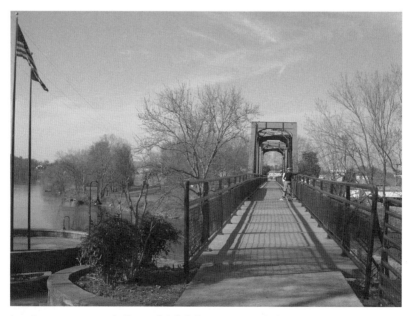

As well as prime river views, the Heritage Park Trail offers access to the Chieftains Museum, a National Historic Landmark.

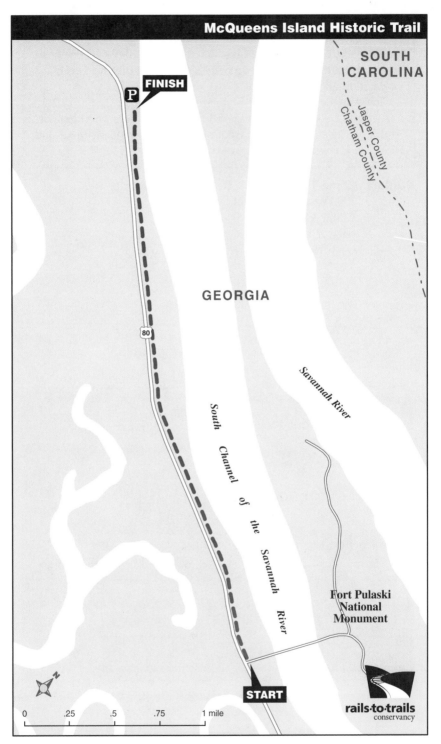

McQueens Island Historic Trail

SOUTH CAROLINA

Jasper County
Chatham County

P FINISH

GEORGIA

80

Savannah River

South Channel of the Savannah River

Fort Pulaski National Monument

START

N

0   .25   .5   .75   1 mile

rails·to·trails
conservancy

McQueens Island Historic Trail

Built on a three-mile stretch of the Savannah & Atlantic Railroad line, the McQueens Island Historic Trail offers a salt-air excursion for nature lovers and history buffs alike. Built in 1887, the railroad carried passengers from Savannah to Tybee Island, a popular turn-of-the-century beach resort. A highway to the island was built in 1923, leading to the demise of the railroad.

From its trailhead just 15 miles east of town, the trail parallels the South Channel of the Savannah River, a major shipping route and entry point to the Port of Savannah. (The trail was six miles long until the wakes of larger ships washed out its western half; plans to rebuild are under way.) Short bridges spirit you across saltwater marshes. Cord grass, cabbage palms, yaupon holly, and coastal cedars line this beautiful trail, and interpretive signs list the native wildlife, including the eastern box turtle, American alligator, diamond back terrapin, bobcat, osprey, red-tailed hawk, and brown pelican. Be on the lookout for these, as well as dolphins frolicking in the river. Conveniently placed benches allow visitors to pause, take in the scenery, and picnic.

Endpoints
Savannah to Fort
Pulaski

Mileage
3

**Roughness
Index**
2

Surface
Gravel

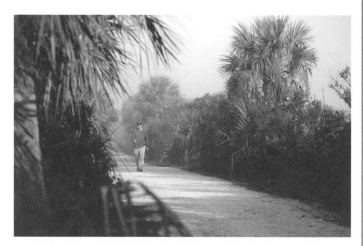

Cabbage palms and the South Channel of the Savannah River line this rail-trail dating back to 1887.

This region boasts an interesting and extensive history, from its earliest inhabitants (Gaulle Indians, followed by early colonists) to the Revolutionary and Civil War battles fought on its soil. Cap your trek with a visit to the massive brick Fort Pulaski, captured in 1862 by Union troops with an experimental rifled cannon. If time permits, head over to Tybee Island, a few miles east of the trail. Tybee's 1732 lighthouse is Georgia's oldest and tallest.

DIRECTIONS

To reach the eastern trailhead, follow US Highway 80 east toward Tybee Island. The trailhead entrance is about 15 miles east of Savannah near a sign for Fort Pulaski National Monument. Parking is available along the road or at the fort.

To reach the western trailhead, follow the directions above, but continue a few miles along US Highway 80 and look for a small roadside parking area just before the turnoff for Fort Pulaski.

Contact: Chatham County Public Works
& Park Services Department
P.O. Box 8161
Savannah, GA 31412
(912) 652-6780
www.chathamcounty.org/pwps_mcqueen.html

Moultrie Trail

In deep south Georgia, Moultrie is a small city with big Southern pride. Billing itself as the "City of Southern Living," Moultrie boasts a thriving agricultural industry, historic homes and commercial buildings, and a state-of-the-art athletic center. Its centerpiece is this 7.5-mile rail-trail, as varied as the city it traverses. In a matter of miles, the Moultrie Trail (a.k.a. Tom "Babe" White Linear Park) will whisk you from woodlands to streetscapes or from a quiet cemetery to a busy restaurant.

Following an old CSX rail bed, the trail leads from downtown Moultrie past a recreation complex and a middle school, through a residential area, and past a country club. You'll cross US Highway 319 before emerging at Moultrie Municipal Airport.

As well as providing excellent recreational space, the trail is a viable and valued transportation corridor with a variety of access points. Williams Middle School students use the trail as a route to school; high school football fans park a few blocks away and walk to games via the trail, and Colquitt Regional Medical Center patients and staff also use the trail.

Endpoints
First Avenue to Moultrie Municipal Airport

Mileage
7.5

Roughness Index
1

Surface
Asphalt, concrete

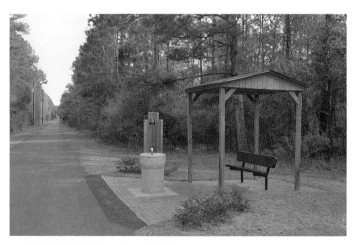

The Moultrie Trail follows a former CSX line.

Moultrie Trail

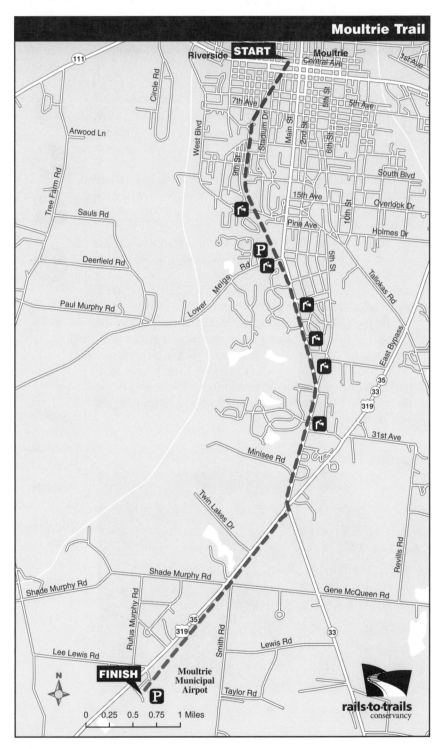

DIRECTIONS

The main trailhead is downtown at the intersection of GA 37/West Central Avenue and First Street NW. Park at the adjacent Wesley Ballpark at First Street NW and First Avenue NW.

To reach the Lower Meigs Road trailhead, take US Highway 319/GA 33/GA 35 (East Bypass) to US Highway 319 Business, which becomes Main Street. Drive north about two miles and turn left on Lower Meigs. Trailhead parking is 100 yards ahead on the right.

To reach the Moultrie Municipal Airport trailhead, take US Highway 319/GA 133/GA 35 (East Bypass) to Airport Drive. Minimal parking is available at the airport, though it's not officially designated as trail parking.

The trail is also accessible via Williams Middle School (1000 Stadium Drive) and the adjacent Jim Buck Goff Recreation Complex.

Contact: City of Moultrie
P.O. Box 3368
Moultrie, GA 31776
(229) 985-1974
www.moultriega.com

Silver Comet Trail

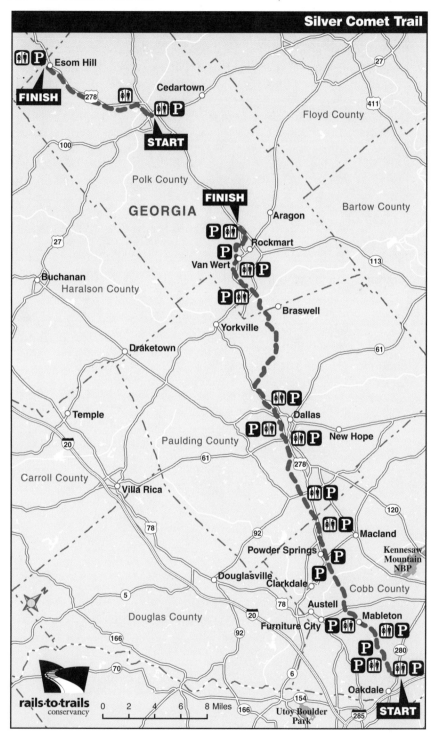

Silver Comet Trail

The Silver Comet Trail follows the bed of the old Seaboard Air Line. From 1947 to 1969, the shiny Silver Comet passenger train provided luxury service between New York City and Birmingham, Alabama. Today, three trestles and a railroad tunnel integrated into the trail design hint at past glories.

The well-maintained 50-mile trail (60 when complete) boasts a 12-foot-wide paved path with mile markers and accommodates nearly all trail uses. An adjacent equestrian path stretches some 40 miles west from Florence Road in Powder Springs. Rounding out the stats are 17 wheelchair-accessible access points (six with horse trailer parking), 15 restrooms, 10 water fountains, and a variety of trailside services.

Today's Silver Comet runs from Smyrna, about 13 miles northwest of Atlanta, through three counties to the Alabama state line. Thirty-eight miles connect Smyrna and Rockmart, followed by an eight-mile gap in the trail. You'll need to navigate back roads to rejoin the route at a restored train depot in tiny Cedartown. From there it's a straight shot to Esom Hill.

The eastern section runs through residential areas, including housing developments with private trail

Endpoints
Smyrna to
Esom Hill

Mileage
50

**Roughness
Index**
1

Surface
Concrete

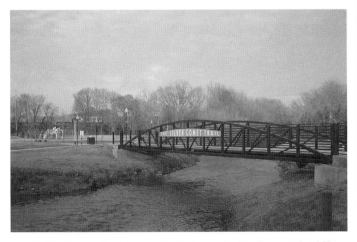

The Silver Comet is Georgia's gem rail-trail featuring railroad trestles, a tunnel, and 50 miles of paved playground.

access. The western section is more bucolic, a mixed landscape of pine stands and farmland. At dusk, the countryside comes alive with animal sounds.

Trail highlights include several relics of its railroading past. At Mile Marker 23, the Pumpkinville Creek Trestle stands 100 feet high and 700 feet long. Standing atop the trestle, you can almost picture the Comet streaking past in a silver blur. At Mile Marker 30.8, the Brushy Mountain Tunnel sounds a spooky note with 700 feet of damp, dark corridor.

You'll find the Silver Comet Depot, a trailside bike rental shop, on Floyd Road in Mableton, while Mile Marker 37.6 heralds your arrival in idyllic, small-town Rockmart. Two miles west of town, baseball and recreation fields provide further entertainment. Cedartown features a restored train depot, as well as places to load up on refreshments for the round-trip to Smyrna.

Plans are underway to link this trail with Alabama's 32-mile Chief Ladiga Trail (see p. 11). The completed network will stretch a whopping 101 miles. In the meantime, the Silver Comet offers a wide array of activities. Its rich history appeals to railroad enthusiasts, and its first-rate facilities draw recreation seekers from miles around. Whether you want to run five miles or bike 50, this rail-trail is an excellent option. Enjoy it for an hour or make an entire day of it.

DIRECTIONS

The Atlanta side of the Silver Comet provides two trailheads: the unofficial Silver Comet Connector trailhead and the official Mavell Road trailhead.

To reach the Silver Comet Connector trailhead, take I-285/Route 407 to Exit 15/Route 280/South Cobb Drive. Head north on South Cobb, turn left on Cumberland Parkway SE, then right on Gaylor Street. The mile-long trailhead is near the shopping complex.

To reach the Mavell Road trailhead, follow the above directions to South Cobb Drive. On South Cobb, continue north, turn left on Cooper Lake Road, then left on Mavell to the trailhead.

To reach the Esom Hill trailhead, take US Highway 278 west. Near Mile Marker 1, turn south on Hardin Road. The trailhead is a half-mile up on the right.

Parking is available at all trailheads.

Contact: The Path Foundation
P.O. Box 14327
(404) 875-7284
www.pathfoundation.org

Simms Mountain Trail

A rugged trek through the North Georgia mountains, this 4.5-mile trail is ideally suited to hikers and mountain bikers. Despite its quiet, dense forest setting, the Simms Mountain Trail does pass several houses, so keep an eye out for local dogs guarding their property.

From the Huffaker Road trailhead, the trail traverses a wooden bridge over a pristine brook broken by waterfalls. Within a quarter mile you'll cross Big Texas Valley Road, though traffic is sparse in this rural area. Here the trail merges with the Georgia Pinhoti Trail, the state's longest footpath.

Over the next mile you'll find evidence of the region's active logging industry off the south side of the trail. Keep trekking west to more remote and scenic sections, where pine forests and dense foliage stretch south to distant mountains, presenting a gorgeous prospect.

While this trail ends at the Chattooga/Floyd county line, if you're feeling adventurous and have the energy, the Georgia Pinhoti Trail continues another 95 miles north. Simply cross the street (GA 100/Holland Road) and continue trekking into the mountains.

Endpoints
Huffaker Road to Chattooga/Floyd county line

Mileage
4.5

Roughness Index
3

Surface
Crushed stone, gravel, dirt, sand

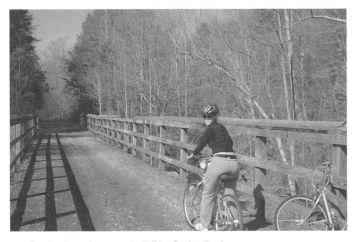
Bicyclists begin their trip at the Huffaker Road trailhead.

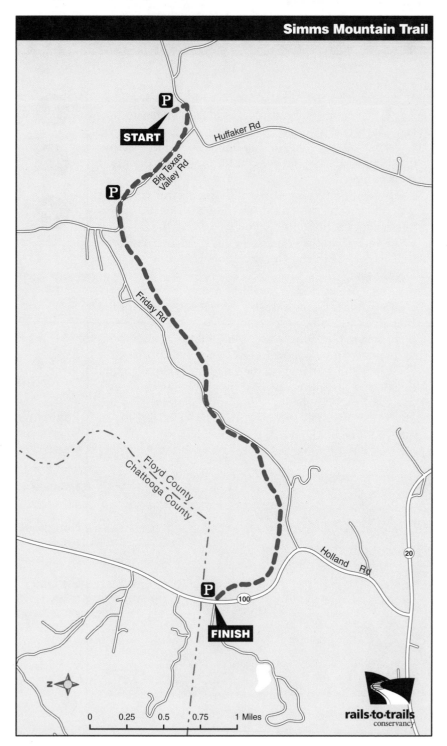

P

START

Huffaker Rd

P

Big Texas Valley Rd

Friday Rd

Floyd County
Chattooga County

Holland Rd

20

P

100

FINISH

Z

0   0.25   0.5   0.75   1 Miles

rails·to·trails
conservancy

DIRECTIONS

For a slightly uphill challenge, start at Huffaker Road. The trailhead can be tricky to find. To reach it from Rome, head west about 10 miles on GA 20 and turn right on Huffaker Road. (Note: Huffaker intersects with GA 20 twice; if you're westbound, turn right the second time it appears). Several miles farther, just past Big Texas Valley Road on the left, you'll reach the unmarked trailhead, also on the left.

To reach the Chattooga/Floyd county line trailhead, continue west on GA 20, turn right on GA 100/Holland Road, and travel several miles north to the county line. A crosswalk and pedestrian road sign mark the trailhead.

Limited parking is available at each trailhead and along Big Texas Valley Road.

Contact: Rome-Floyd Parks & Recreation Authority
300 West Third Street
Rome, GA 30162
(706) 291-0766
www.rfpra.com

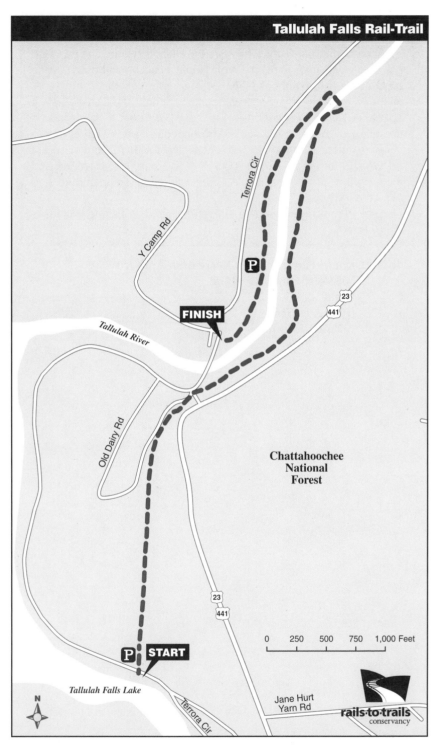

Tallulah Falls Rail-Trail

Terrora Cir

Y Camp Rd

P

FINISH

Tallulah River

23
441

Old Dairy Rd

Chattahoochee
National
Forest

23
441

0   250   500   750   1,000 Feet

P   START

Tallulah Falls Lake

Terrora Cir

N

Jane Hurt
Yarn Rd

rails·to·trails
conservancy

Tallulah Falls Rail-Trail

The Tallulah Falls Rail-Trail (a.k.a. Shortline Trail) spins a short, smooth circuit through Tallulah Gorge State Park. From its trailhead beside Tallulah Falls Lake, the 1.7-mile paved path meanders through a beautiful southern Appalachian forest and crosses a small suspension bridge over the Tallulah River. You can ride out and back or combine the trail with a short road segment to form a loop.

The route follows the easy grade of the old Tallulah Falls Railway, a great alternative to more arduous hiking trails that scale the nearly 1,000-foot granite walls of Tallulah Gorge. In the late 19th century the railroad granted tourists access to the gorge and its spectacular waterfalls. While you can't see the chasm from the trail, a detour across US Highway 23/441 will take you to its dizzying lip.

In the spring and fall, controlled releases from Tallulah Dam bring kayakers intent on challenging the imposing river, while Halloween heralds the annual Wails to Trails event, when costumed hikers haunt the trail.

Endpoints
Within Tallulah
Gorge State Park

Mileage
1.7

**Roughness
Index**
1

Surface
Asphalt

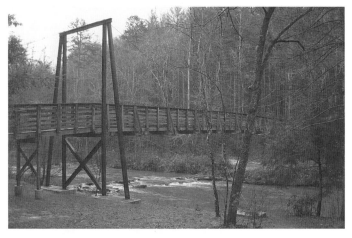
A suspension bridge crosses the Tallulah River.

DIRECTIONS

Tallulah Gorge State Park is on US Highway 23/441 in North Georgia, just north of the town of Tallulah Falls. To reach it from town, drive north about a half mile and turn left at the first park entrance, just past the dam. Continue along the park road to the Shortline Trail parking lot ($4 per car). The trail lies just south of the main park entrance.

Contact: Tallulah Gorge State Park
338 Jane Hurt Drive
Tallulah Falls, GA 30573
(800) 864-7275
www.gastateparks.org

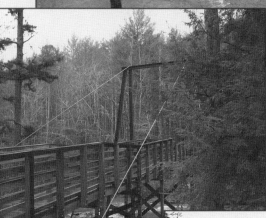

The Tallulah Falls Rail-Trail is a strikingly scenic path contained within Tallulah Gorge State Park.

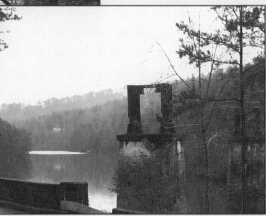

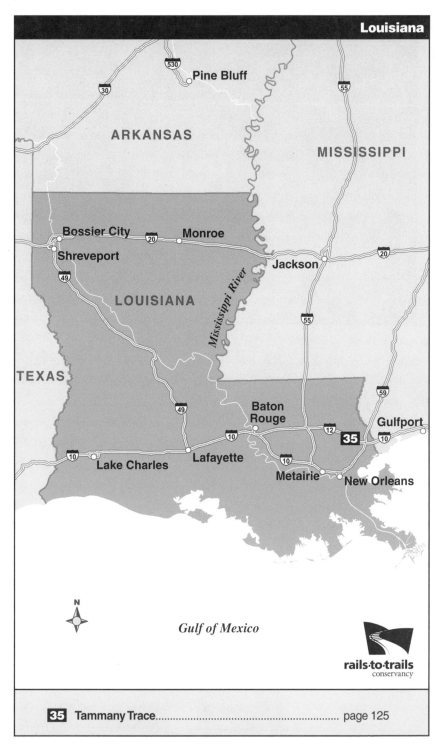

Louisiana

530
Pine Bluff
30
55

ARKANSAS

MISSISSIPPI

Bossier City
20
Monroe
Shreveport
49

Jackson
20

LOUISIANA

Mississippi River

55

TEXAS

49

Baton
Rouge
10
12
35
Gulfport
59
10

10
Lake Charles
Lafayette
10
Metairie
New Orleans

N

Gulf of Mexico

rails·to·trails
conservancy

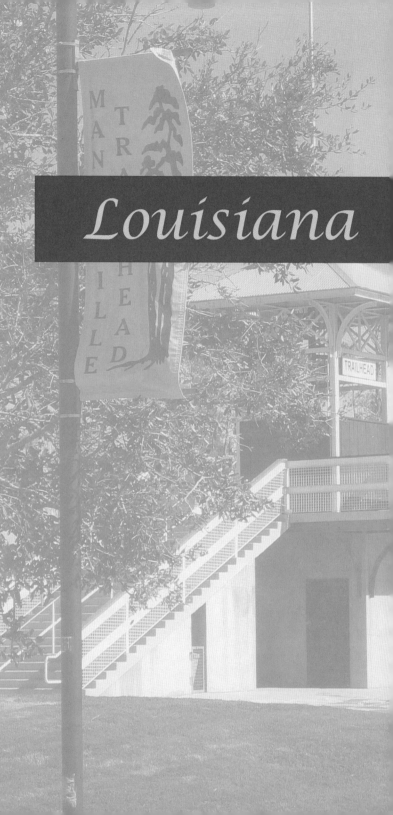

Louisiana

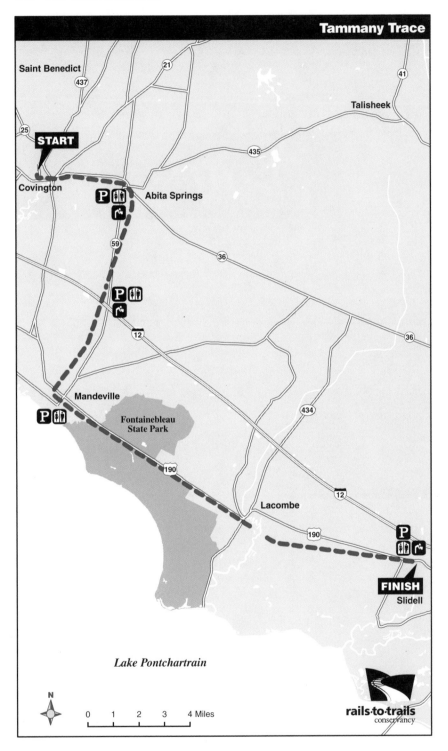

Tammany Trace

Saint Benedict

437

21

41

Talisheek

25

START

435

Covington

P

Abita Springs

59

36

P

12

36

Mandeville

Fontainebleau
State Park

434

190

12

Lacombe

190

P

FINISH
Slidell

Lake Pontchartrain

N

0   1   2   3   4 Miles

rails·to·trails
conservancy

Tammany Trace

On the north shore of Lake Pontchartrain, Tammany Trace offers a fascinating, scenic trek through five St. Tammany Parish communities. Before the 24-mile causeway was completed in the 1960s, this area was quite cut off from the sway of New Orleans. Today, the parish is one of the fastest growing in the state. Despite the rapid growth, however, this 27.5-mile corridor remains blessed with beautiful views of woods and wetlands.

Passing through the historic towns of Covington, Abita Springs, and Mandeville, you'll experience the piney woods and moss-draped oaks that earned the area its Ozone Belt nickname. In the late 1800s New Orleanians seeking respite from the oppressive heat of the coastal plain chose this as a vacation spot. Today, the trail passes many of their stately retreats.

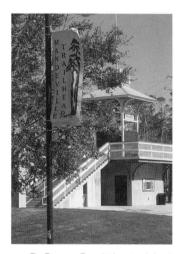

The Tammany Trace bridges trendy local neighborhoods and famous Louisiana swampland in its 27.5 miles of paved trail.

While the western endpoint is in trendy Covington, the first trailhead (with parking, restrooms, and water fountains) lies seven miles east in Abita Springs. The latter is also home to the famed Abita Brewpub, which serves a pleasant lunch at trailside seating (park at adjacent Abita Springs Park). The famous local beer and root beer are brewed nearby.

The route south to Mandeville threads a mostly suburban setting with several street crossings. Beware the problematic crossing at US Highway 190; plans call for improvements by 2008. To connect with local culture, stop by the Saturday morning market at the Mandeville trailhead to browse handmade items and sample a variety of local foods.

Endpoints
Covington, Mandeville, Lacombe, and Slidell

Mileage
27.5

Roughness Index
1

Surface
Asphalt

Beyond Mandeville, the trail leads southeast through the damp, heavy wetlands climate. This is the Louisiana of Deep South lore. You'll come within several blocks of Lake Pontchartrain before angling inland toward the bayou. Keep watch for alligators, as well as the nefarious nutria, a semiaquatic rodent that's been gnawing its way through the Louisiana wetlands since the 1930s.

Though Hurricane Katrina did ravage the trail—not to mention the rest of southeast Louisiana, crews have removed the fallen trees, and most of the route is again open. That said, Katrina did push back plans to improve trail access, particularly along the Mandeville–Slidell section.

Another impediment is an unfinished bridge across the Lacombe Bayou on the eastern trail section. The route currently stops at Lake Road to the west and South Oaklawn Drive to the east. While cyclists can bypass this gap via US Highway 190, the high volume of traffic makes this detour hazardous. Plans call for construction of a new bridge across the bayou by the end of 2008.

DIRECTIONS

To reach the Tammany Trace trailhead, take I-12 east to LA 59 north, cross Little Creek, and turn left on Koop Drive. Rangers staff a visitor center in a green caboose past the St. Tammany Parish government building. Park beside the caboose.

Contact: Tammany Trace
21490 Koop Drive
Mandeville, LA 70471
(985) 867-9490
www.tammanytrace.org

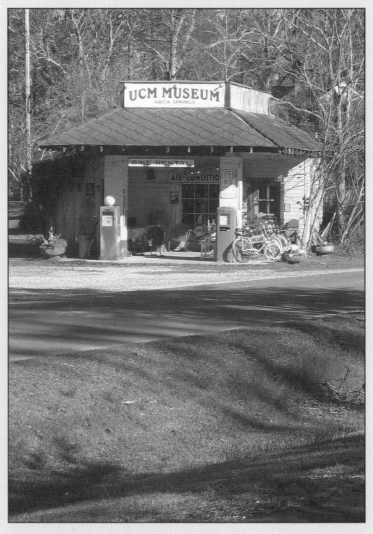

Trailside amenities make a trip on the Trace even more of a treat.

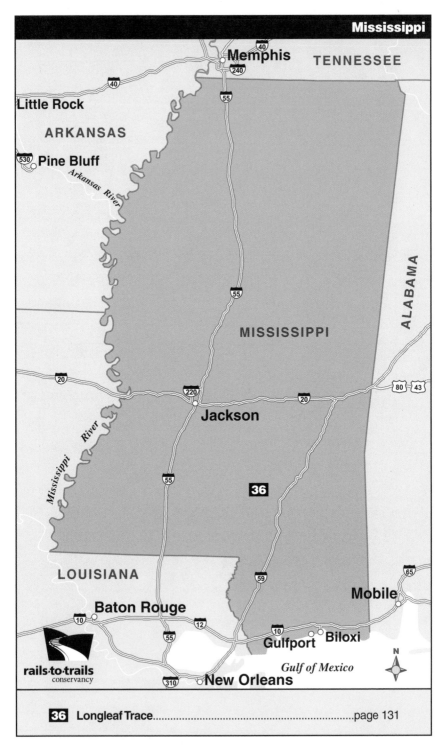

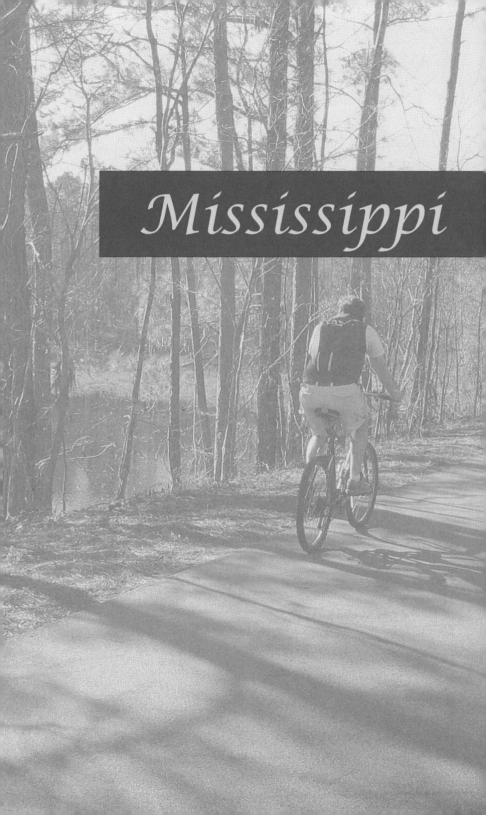

Mississippi

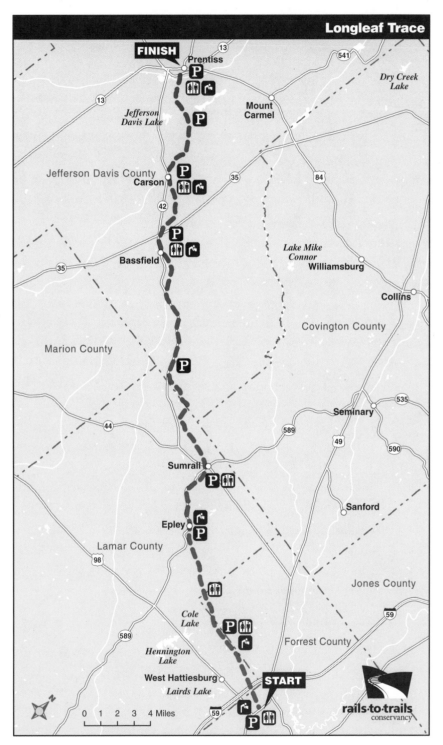

Longleaf Trace

Stretching 41 miles northwest from the University of Southern Mississippi (Southern Miss) in Hattiesburg to small-town Prentiss, Longleaf Trace traverses landscapes that range from the bustling heart of Mississippi's third-largest city to the rural farmland that predominates in this area.

A designated National Recreation Trail, the trace is the longest rail-trail in the south-central U.S. It runs atop a stretch of Mississippi Central Railroad line that saw much activity as the region's timber industry flourished between the late 1800s and 1920s. As the industry began to fade, so too did the need for the rail service, and although the railroad struggled on into the 1970s, it eventually ceased to be economically viable. Fortunately, a concerted effort by local groups and individuals preserved the corridor, and in 2000 it opened as a trail.

Today the route is again active, as cyclists, inline skaters, and pedestrians ply the trail's smooth, well-maintained surface. Eight small covered rest areas along the route provide travelers with shade, restrooms, and vending machines, while three small shelters offer places to wait out brief summer rain showers.

Endpoints
Hattiesburg to Prentiss

Mileage
41

Roughness Index
1

Surface
Asphalt

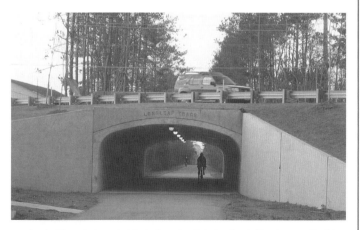

Longleaf Trace designers had the trail user in mind when they built underpasses like this one to allow users to avoid tangling with traffic.

Start your trip at the trace gateway on the Southern Miss campus, where welcome center staff can offer advice, provide maps, and help visitors identify the many tree species that line the route, including the namesake longleaf pine. Bike rentals and parking are available here.

Over the first few miles, the trail negotiates several tunnels and bridges. Leaving Hattiesburg behind, you'll progress through a range of quintessentially Southern landscapes, from piney woods and wetlands to small lakes and charming towns. Fifteen miles northwest, in Epley, the trail meets a dirt equestrian path that zigzags across the trace some 25 miles to Carson.

Thirty-three miles out, just past Bassfield, is a stable, while two miles farther is a primitive camping site. The rolling hills that define this section may pose a challenge to less experienced cyclists. While the grades aren't particularly steep, factor them in if you're on a day trip or traveling with small children.

At trail's end in downtown Prentiss, an attractive trailhead provides restrooms, parking, and vending machines. If you've chosen to end your trip in Hattiesburg instead, consider renting a canoe and plunging into Black Creek, a National Scenic River about 10 miles south of the Southern Miss gateway. Like the trace itself, the creek will take you for a gentle, slow-moving ramble through central Mississippi's piney woods.

DIRECTIONS

To reach the Hattiesburg gateway, take I-59 to Exit 65/Hardy Street and head east. Following the brown trail signs, turn left on 38th Avenue, then right at the next light on Fourth Street. Just past the Southern Miss football stadium, turn left into the trailhead parking lot.

To reach the Prentiss trailhead from Hattiesburg, take US Highway 49 about 27 miles northwest to Collins and turn west on US Highway 84. Nearly 20 miles west in Prentiss, the trace crosses the highway near its trailhead in a park. Just shy of this crossing, turn right on Front Street to access the trailhead.

Contact: Pearl and Leaf Rivers Rails-to-Trails Recreational District
2895 West Fourth Street
Hattiesburg, MS 39404
(601) 450-5247
www.longleaftrace.org

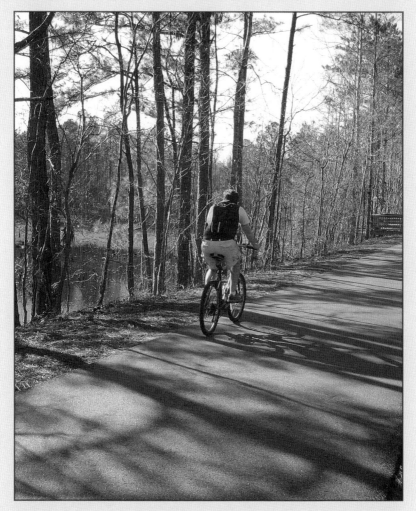

Within minutes of leaving the busy University of Southern Mississippi and crossing beneath I-59, you'll find yourself in truly remote southern Mississippi wilderness.

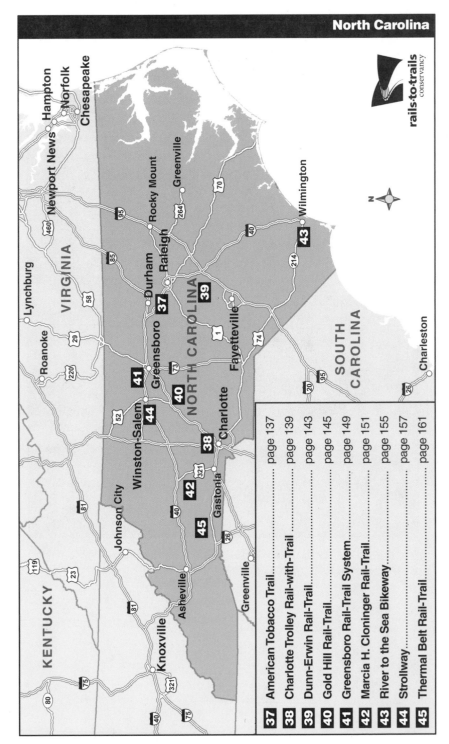

rails·to·trails
conservancy

North Carolina

DOWN
TOWN

LINCOLNTON

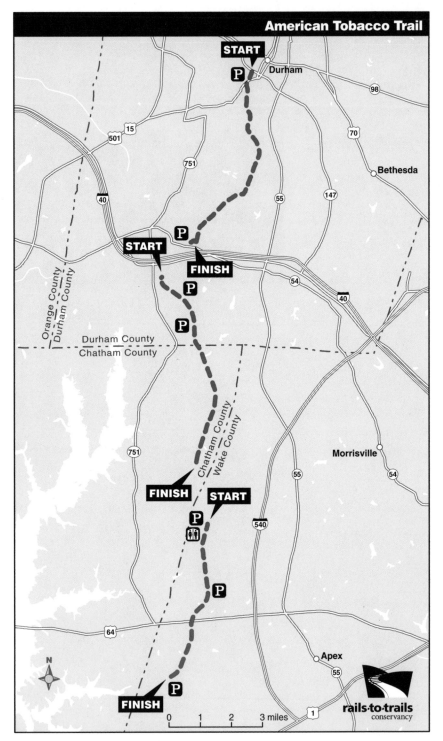

American Tobacco Trail

START
P
Durham
98
15
501
751
70
Bethesda
40
55
147
P
START
FINISH
54
P
40
P
Orange County
Durham County
Durham County
Chatham County
751
Chatham County
Wake County
Morrisville
54
55
FINISH
START
P
540
P
64
55
Apex
P
FINISH
55
1

0   1   2   3 miles

rails·to·trails
conservancy

American Tobacco Trail

Someday the American Tobacco Trail will extend uninterrupted from Durham 22 miles south through Chatham County to Wake County. For now, visitors can access about 18 miles of open trail in three disconnected segments (identified here as northern, middle, and southern). Each segment sports a different surface, enabling a variety of uses.

The 6.5-mile northern segment, with a well-maintained asphalt surface, is a favorite among inline skaters and cyclists. Starting from the Durham Bulls Athletic Park, this urban pathway winds through neighborhoods and up behind the Southpoint Crossing Shopping Center to its current end at Highway 54.

Starting from Massey Chapel Road south of I-40, the 6.2-mile middle segment runs south on a dirt, grass, and gravel track through neighborhoods and piney woods into Chatham County. The maintained stretch ends at New Hope Church Road, though mountain bikers can test the rough paths beyond either endpoint. Undecked trestles across Northeast and Panther creeks are scheduled for completion, and a pedestrian bridge will eventually span I-40 and link up with the northern segment. This segment and the southern segment are open to equestrians.

Endpoints
Durham Bulls
Athletic Park to
New Hill–Olive
Chapel Road

Mileage
18

**Roughness
Index**
2

Surface
Asphalt, ballast,
gravel, grass, dirt

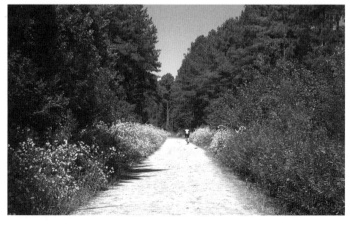

Wildflowers decorate the American Tobacco Trail in the summer months.

Running from White Oak Church Road to New Hill-Olive Chapel Road in Wake County, the 5.3-mile southern segment follows a ballast track through beautiful pines. Trailside amenities include dedicated parking and information kiosks with trail brochures and maps. A segment leading north to the Chatham County line is set to open soon.

The ATT's rural sections boast plentiful wildlife, including beavers, herons, hawks, songbirds, vultures, squirrels, owls, and deer. While hunters use the middle and southern segments to access wildlife areas, they are not allowed to carry loaded firearms on the trail.

When the trail is complete, users will be able to ride or walk from urban environs through the suburbs to a surprisingly rural setting. In the meantime, each segment holds its own charms. Choose Durham for a smooth cycle amid the city bustle. For rural bliss, head south to Wake. And if you're searching for that happy medium, the middle segment south of I-40 is for you.

DIRECTIONS

To reach the northern trailhead, head south on US 15/501 Business/North Roxboro Street; this will turn into South Mangum Street. At West Pettigrew Street, turn right, followed by a left on Blackwell Street. Parking is available beneath the East-West Expressway on Morehead Avenue, across from the Durham Bulls Athletic Park. Trail parking is also available at Solite Park off Fayetteville Street and at Southpoint Crossing Shopping Center, just north of I-40 at the intersection of Fayetteville and NC 54.

To reach the middle trailhead, take I-40 to Exit 276 and head south on Fayetteville Street. Two miles down, turn left on Scott King Road. A parking lot is being built just west of the trailhead; until it opens, park on the shoulder beneath the power lines. A smaller lot is being built on the west side of Fayetteville Road, just north of a bridge across the trail. Steps will provide access.

To reach the southern trailhead from Raleigh, take US Highway 1 south to Exit 89 toward New Hill/Jordan Lake, turn right, and drive about four miles up New Hill–Olive Chapel Road. Trailhead parking is on the right. To reach the other access point, take US Highway 64 west, turn right on Jenks Road, then left on Wimberley Road. Parking is on the right.

Contact: Triangle Rails-to-Trails Conservancy
P.O. Box 61091
Durham, NC 27715
(919) 545-9104
www.triangletrails.org

Charlotte Trolley Rail-with-Trail

Take a trip down memory lane by strolling or cycling the Charlotte Trolley Rail-with-Trail. This two-mile cement trail follows the Charlotte Trolley as it tootles its way from Ninth Street in Uptown to Tremont Avenue in the historic South End.

The original trolley line closed in 1938. Luckily, a University of North Carolina history professor was able to track down the last trolley—No. 85, and this piece of history is now back in service on the rail-with-trail, along with three replica trolleys.

As the trail traverses the city streets from Uptown, it passes the popular ImaginOn children's learning center and Charlotte Bobcats Arena before leading directly through the Charlotte Convention Center. If the center is closed or you're biking the route, you must go around the block (right on East Second, left on South College, then left on East Stonewall), then either climb the stairs or take the elevator in a parking garage across the street to rejoin the trail.

The South End hosts both the Charlotte Trolley barn and museum at Atherton Mill, as well as the popular South End Gallery Crawl, held the first Friday of each month by trailside art galleries.

Endpoints
Ninth Street to
Tremont Avenue

Mileage
2

Roughness Index
1

Surface
Concrete

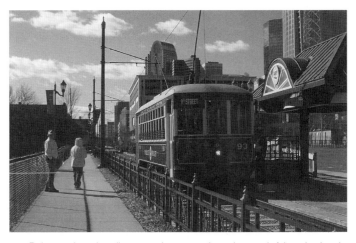

Trail users admire the trolley cars as they pass on the northwest end of this rail-with-trail.

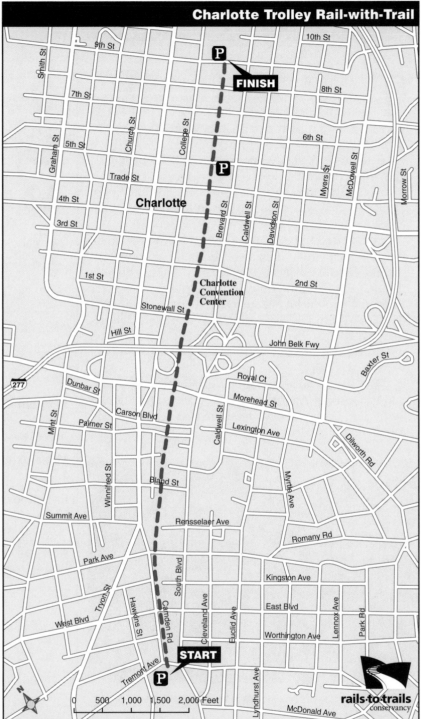

Charlotte Trolley Rail-with-Trail

The entire route is fairly well marked, and trash receptacles, benches, bike stands, and streetlights line the way. And once you've walked the trail in one direction, you can catch the trolley back.

DIRECTIONS

In downtown Charlotte, the trolley line runs south from East Ninth Street between College and Brevard to just past East Tremont Avenue in the South End. Parking lots line the route. If you choose the lot at East Ninth Street, park toward the back and not in the spaces reserved for the fire department.

Contact: Charlotte Center City Partners
128 South Tryon Street, Suite 1960
Charlotte, NC 28202
(888) 424-2756
www.charlottecentercity.org

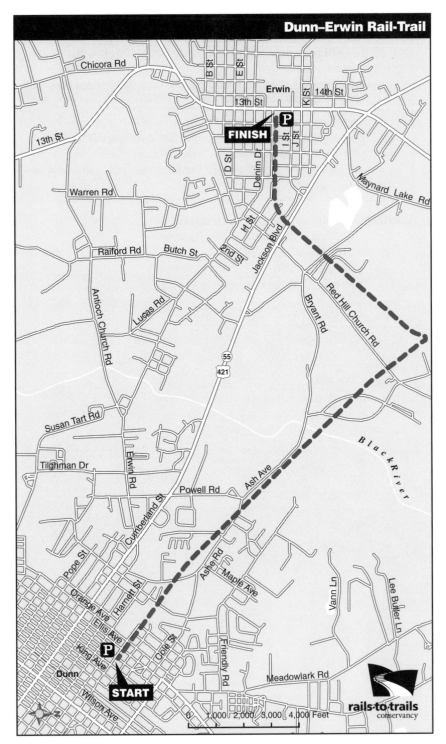

Dunn–Erwin Rail-Trail

Dunn–Erwin Rail-Trail

A memorial at the Erwin trailhead of the Dunn–Erwin Rail-Trail reads, TO THE PIONEER MEN AND WOMEN WHO LABORED IN THE FIELDS AND COTTON MILLS AND ESTABLISHED THE TOWN OF DUKE, WHICH BECAME ERWIN ON JAN. 1, 1926. And as you ride or walk the 5.3 miles between these rural towns, you can almost picture workers hunched over in the cotton rows. The trail also crosses the beautiful Black River and traverses wetlands and woodlands.

Students at North Carolina State University created the trail master plan in 2001, seeking to connect neighborhoods, schools, commercial districts, and two downtowns, while also promoting the area's rural heritage and protecting the sensitive habitat that surrounds the corridor. The result is a wonderful, safe route for recreation, exercise, and exposure to rural America.

While the current surface is gravel, the Dunn–Erwin Trail Authority hopes to one day pave the trail. If wheelchair users are comfortable using their wheelchairs on gravel, the road-level route is otherwise accessible. Nearby attractions include parks, the Cape Fear River, the Erwin History Room, the General Lee Airborne Museum, the Averasboro Battlefield Museum, and the Centennial Trail in downtown Erwin.

Endpoints
Dunn to Erwin

Mileage
5.3

Roughness Index
2

Surface
Gravel

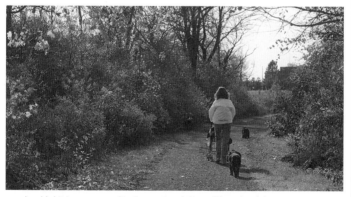

Local habitat was preserved in the creation of this useful, rural trail that connects homes, businesses, and schools.

143

DIRECTIONS FROM THE NORTH

To reach the Dunn trailhead, take I-95 south to Exit 73, head west on Cumberland Street/US Highway 421/NC 55, then turn right on Orange Avenue. Drive three blocks to Harnett Street and park along the road or in the Harnett Primary School lot. The trailhead is behind the school.

To reach the Erwin trailhead, continue on US Highway 421/NC 55 past Dunn. In Erwin, turn left on Old Field Church Road, then right on East H Street. The trail ends in the median on this street.

Contact: Dunn Area Tourism Authority
P.O. Box 310
Dunn, NC 28335
(910) 892-3282
www.dunntourism.org/attractions.asp

Gold Hill Rail-Trail

A trip along the Gold Hill Rail-Trail through this historic village will transport you back to a time when North Carolina was the country's only gold-producing state. Signs posted every few hundred feet along the mile-long dirt and gravel path detail the history of mining in the state. While gold was unofficially discovered here in 1799 by a 12-year-old boy, in its glory days Gold Hill was the richest mining property east of the Mississippi.

The trail begins about 100 yards past the junction of St. Stephens Church Road and Baptist Church Road. There's no sign or even a clear path to indicate that the strip of grass along the road is a trail, but if you want the full history lesson, park at St. Stephen's and backtrack to this point. On the route back to your car, you'll pass the old Randolph Shaft, a miner's field, the powder house, and the assay office, where miners staked their claims and weighed their gold. Just past the assay office is the first historical marker. Cross the street here to join the clearly defined gravel trail.

Endpoints
Gold Hill to
Cabarrus
County line

Mileage
1

**Roughness
Index**
2

Surface
Gravel, dirt

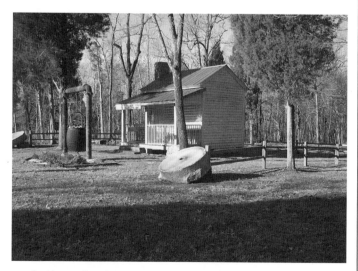

An old assay office where miners staked their claim and weighed their gold has been preserved on the Gold Hill Rail-Trail.

145

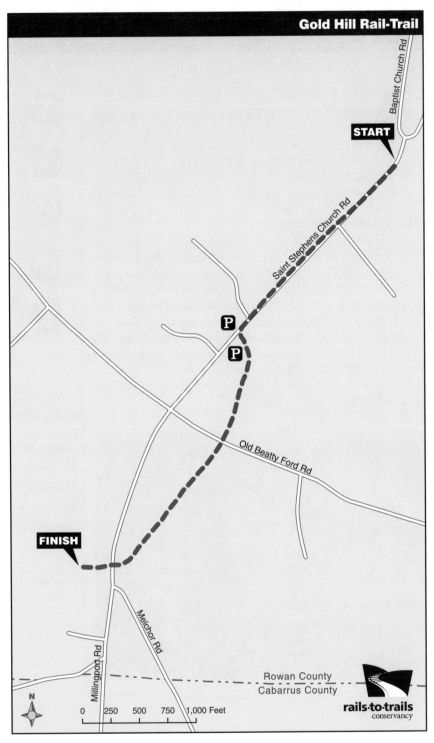

Gold Hill Rail-Trail

Much of the onward trail passes through forest, so keep watch for such wildlife as deer and broadtail hawks. There are a few swampy patches, so be prepared for a muddy trek if you visit following a rainstorm. Back in the village, check out the various historic buildings that have been restored as cafés, antique shops, and museums.

DIRECTIONS

Take I-85 to Exit 76 and head south on US Highway 52. In Gold Hill, turn right at the post office on Doby Drive, a quick left on Old US Highway 80 and a quick right on St. Stephens Church Road. Park at St. Stephen's Church or in the small lot across the road. The trailhead lies back up the road, just shy of the St. Stephens Church/Baptist Church intersection.

Contact: Historic Gold Hill & Mines Foundation
P.O. Box 206
Gold Hill, NC 28071
(704) 267-9439
www.historicgoldhill.com

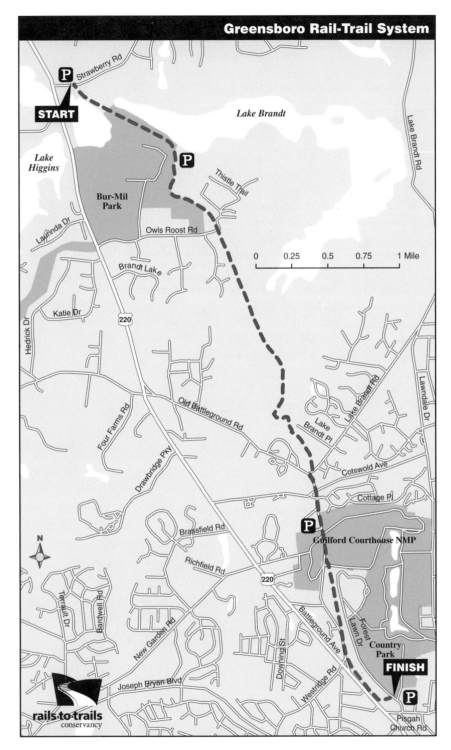

Greensboro Rail-Trail System

Strawberry Rd

START

Lake Brandt

Lake Brandt Rd

Lake Higgins

Thistle Trail

Bur-Mil Park

Laurinda Dr

Owls Roost Rd

0   0.25   0.5   0.75   1 Mile

Brandt Lake

Hedrick Dr

Katie Dr

220

Old Battleground Rd

Lawndale Dr

Four Farms Rd

Lake Brandt Pl

Lake Brandt Rd

Drawbridge Pky

Cotswold Ave

Cottage Pl

Brassfield Rd

Guilford Courthouse NMP

Richfield Rd

220

Terrault Dr

Bardwell Rd

New Garden Rd

Dowling St

Battleground Ave

Westridge Rd

Forest Lawn Dr

Country Park

FINISH

Joseph Bryan Blvd

rails·to·trails
conservancy

Pisgah Church Rd

Greensboro Rail-Trail System

Comprising two connecting paths—the 3.4-mile Lake Brandt Greenway and 1.8-mile Bicentennial Greenway—this gentle, scenic rail-trail system will eventually extend north to Summerfield and south to downtown Greensboro. Blending a healthy dose of nature with multiple connections to area parks and walking trails, the route follows the path of the old Atlantic & Yadkin Railway, which reached Greensboro in 1884.

Lake Brandt, Greensboro's oldest and second-largest reservoir, provides an ideal setting for the first leg of your trek. Offering beautiful lake views, the trail winds though a pine and mixed hardwood forest alive with native wildflowers and resident fauna. Pause on any of several bridges, particularly the 140-foot H. Michael Weaver Bridge, to spot such common and migratory birds as bald eagles, blue herons, egrets, and ospreys. Signs mark possible side trips on the Owl's Roost, Palmetto, and Nat Greene trails.

At the intersection of Old Battleground and Lake Brandt roads, the Lake Brandt Greenway merges with the Bicentennial Greenway. This section of the Greensboro Rail-Trail System runs through a residential

Endpoints
Strawberry Road to Pisgah Church Road

Mileage
5.2

Roughness Index
1

Surface
Asphalt, concrete, crushed stone

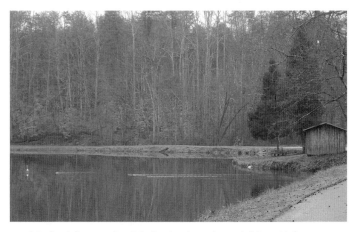

Lake Brandt Greenway skirts Lake Brandt at the northern end of the trail before connecting with the Bicentennial Greenway.

neighborhood and links to Country Park and the adjacent Guilford Courthouse National Military Park.

DIRECTIONS

To reach the Lake Brandt Greenway trailhead, take US Highway 220/Battleground Avenue north and turn right on Strawberry Road. Drive 0.3 mile and turn right into the greenway parking lot.

To reach the southernmost Bicentennial Greenway trailhead, take US Highway 220/Battleground Avenue south and turn left on Pisgah Church Road, followed by an immediate left on Forest Lawn Drive (entrance to Country Park). Parking is available on the west side of the Lewis Recreation Center.

Trail users can access a third trailhead at Bur-Mil Park off Owl's Roost Road, two miles south of Strawberry Road on US Highway 220/Battleground Avenue. Park beside the Frank Sharpe Jr. Wildlife Education Center.

The Bicentennial Greenway and Bur-Mil Park trailheads are wheelchair accessible.

Contact: Greensboro Parks & Recreation
Trails and Greenways Division
Frank Sharpe Jr. Wildlife Education Center
5834 Bur-Mil Club Road
Greensboro, NC 27410
(336) 373-3816
www.greensboro-nc.gov/departments/parks/facilities/
trails/default.htm

Marcia H. Cloninger Rail-Trail

The half-mile Marcia H. Cloninger Rail-Trail, known locally as the Lincolnton Rail-Trail, offers a chance to search the heart of this small Southern town, highlighted by a stately courthouse, model Main Street, thriving arts scene, and nearby lakes and mountains. Once an eyesore covered in kudzu and debris, the former Norfolk Southern Railroad corridor is now the pride and joy of "Lovable Lincolnton."

From the old railroad depot at Pine and North Poplar streets, two blocks north of Main, the trail meanders through town, briefly sharing its corridor with an active railroad line. Expect to encounter both locals and visitors out for exercise or on a break from the specialty and antique shops. The smooth, paved trail is especially popular with inline skaters and parents pushing baby strollers. Benches line the route, inviting you to pause and take in this enchanting town and trail.

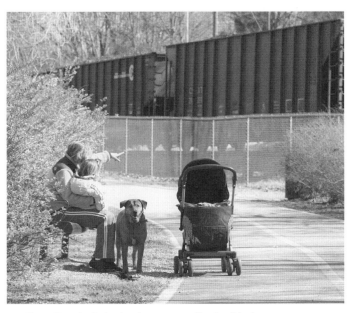

The trail has a brief rail-with-trail segment near Church and Academy streets.

Endpoints
East Pine Street
to West Congress
Street, Lincolnton

Mileage
0.5

**Roughness
Index**
1

Surface
Asphalt

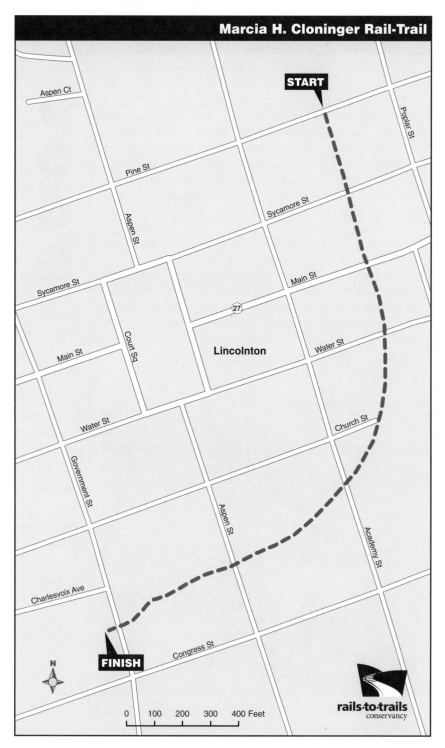

Marcia H. Cloninger Rail-Trail

START

Aspen Ct

Poplar St

Pine St

Sycamore St

Aspen St

Sycamore St

Main St

27

Court Sq

Lincolnton

Water St

Main St

Water St

Church St

Government St

Aspen St

Academy St

Charlesvoix Ave

FINISH

Congress St

N

0   100   200   300   400 Feet

rails-to-trails
conservancy

DIRECTIONS

From Charlotte, take I-85 south to Exit 10 and head north on US Highway 321. Take Exit 24 and follow NC 27/Main Street west into Lincolnton. Turn right on North Poplar Street, and drive one block to the intersection of North Poplar and East Pine. The trailhead is on East Pine, behind the old railroad depot. Street parking is available across from the depot.

Contact: City of Lincolnton Planning Department
P.O. Box 617
Lincolnton, NC 28093
(704) 736-8930
www.ci.lincolnton.nc.us

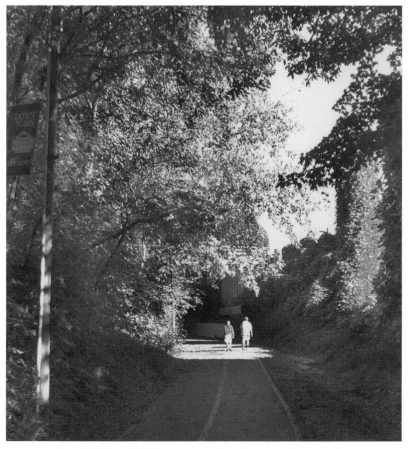

The half-mile Marcia H. Cloninger Rail-Trail is a source of pride for Lincolnton residents.

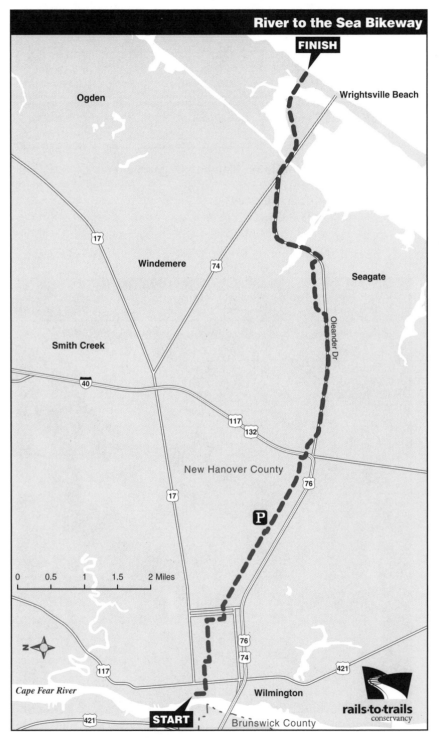

River to the Sea Bikeway

FINISH

Ogden

Wrightsville Beach

17

Windemere

74

Seagate

Smith Creek

Oleander Dr

40

117

132

New Hanover County

76

P

0   0.5   1   1.5   2 Miles

17

76

74

N

117

421

Wilmington

Cape Fear River

START

421

Brunswick County

rails·to·trails
conservancy

River to the Sea Bikeway

Road cyclists who thrive on the adrenaline rush of riding beside an 18-wheeler will love all 11 miles of the River to the Sea Bikeway. But if quiet, traffic-free greenways are more your style, steer over to Colwell Avenue for the two-mile off-road portion of the bikeway.

North Carolina's many bike routes are posted with small signs bearing a picture of a bicycle and the number of the route you're following. The River to the Sea Bikeway is Route 1 and well marked by such signs. Following the historic trolley route to Wrightsville Beach, the bikeway begins beside the Cape Fear River in downtown Wilmington. The off-road, cement greenway begins just off Colwell, nearly two miles into the bikeway, and leads through a residential neighborhood. Merging onto the Park Avenue median, the surface switches to packed sand/dirt, making for an easy ride or walk.

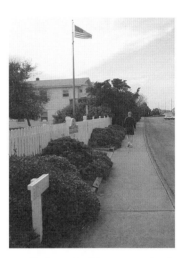

The River to Sea Bikeway is a patchwork quilt of trail and on-road pathways.

If you're following the road route and plan to ride all the way to Johnnie Mercer's Pier in Wrightsville Beach, please note that the sign on Oleander Drive indicating that bicyclists should cross this busy street is not part of the bikeway. Instead, take Oleander out to Wrightsville Avenue, then follow the bike route signs east over the drawbridge and past the Wrightsville Beach visitor center.

Again, the road route is not for the inexperienced or faint of heart, and cyclists with children are particularly advised to limit their excursion to the off-road greenway.

Endpoints
Wilmington to
Wrightsville Beach

Mileage
11

**Roughness
Index**
1

Surface
Asphalt, cement,
sand, dirt

DIRECTIONS

To reach the Wilmington trailhead, take US Highway 74/76 east into Wilmington, turn left on Third Street, then left again on Market Street. The bikeway begins at the end of Market where it meets Water Street.

To reach the off-road section of the route, ride south on Front Street and turn left on Castle Street. After crossing 17th Street, veer right on Colwell Avenue. The greenway is clearly marked with a NO MOTORIZED VEHICLES sign.

There is no dedicated trail parking, but road parking is available.

Contact: Wilmington Urban Area Metropolitan
Planning Organization
P.O. Box 1810
Wilmington, NC 28402
(910) 342-2781
www.wmpo.org

Strollway

A s its name suggests, the Winston-Salem Strollway presents the perfect setting for a leisurely walk. Completed in 1988, the popular rail-trail links Winston-Salem's modern business district with historic Old Salem.

The first segment threads though several engaging downtown blocks and crosses beneath I-40. As you approach the underpass, the cityscape gives way to green spaces, fragrant magnolias, and residential neighborhoods.

A half mile farther you'll reach the Old Salem Visitor Center. If time allows, pop in and explore this restored historic district. Established in 1766 by Moravian craftsmen, it grew into a thriving trading center and reputable source of high-quality handicrafts. Today it's one of the country's most authentic and best documented colonial sites, boasting 100 restored and reconstructed buildings.

A half mile beyond the visitor center, the Strollway ends at West Salem Avenue. If you have the energy, continue east on the connecting Salem Creek Trail, which skirts the creek for three miles and emerges on scenic Salem Lake.

Endpoints
Central business district to Old Salem, Winston-Salem

Mileage
1.2

Roughness Index
1

Surface
Asphalt, crushed stone

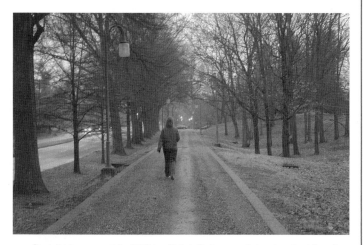

The trail takes you past the Old Salem Visitor's Center, a good place to gather information on this historical town.

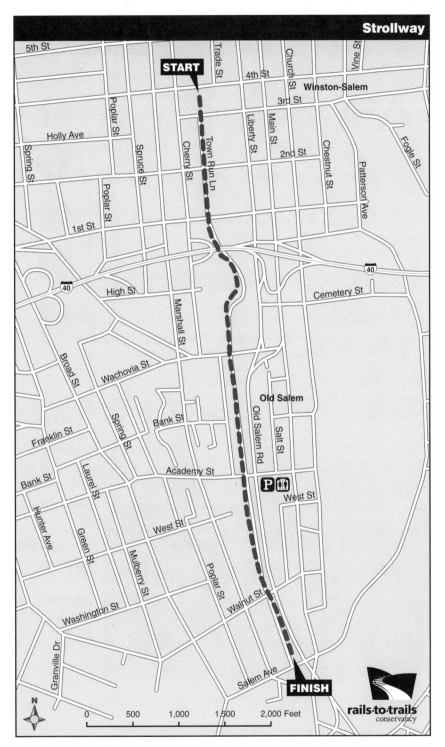

Strollway

START

Winston-Salem

Old Salem

FINISH

rails·to·trails
conservancy

DIRECTIONS

To reach the central business district trailhead, take I-40 Business west to Exit 5C/Cherry Street, head north on Cherry, and turn right on Fourth Street. The trailhead is on Fourth between Cherry and Trade. Limited street parking is available, or you can use the public parking garage on Cherry between Fourth and Fifth.

To reach the West Salem Avenue trailhead from downtown, head south on Liberty Street, which merges with Old Salem Road. The trailhead is just west of the intersection of Old Salem and West Salem. Trail parking is available at the Old Salem Visitor Center (900 Old Salem Road, (888) 653-7253, www.oldsalem.org).

Contact: Winston-Salem Recreation & Parks
P.O. Box 2511
Winston-Salem, NC 27102
(336) 727-2063
www.cityofws.org/recreation/greenways_trails/
greenways_trails.html

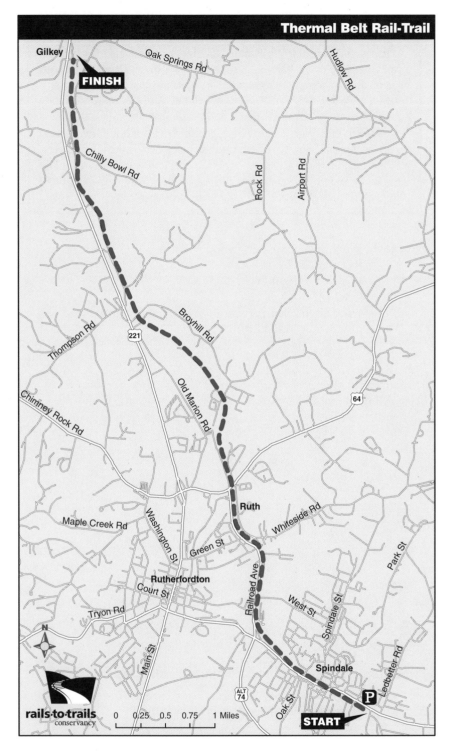

Thermal Belt Rail-Trail

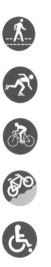

If you enjoy rail-trails that flaunt their railroading past, you're sure to love the Thermal Belt Rail-Trail. This well-maintained route runs eight miles from Spindale north to Gilkey, passing through the equally tiny towns of Rutherfordton and Ruth. Its crushed stone surface barely disguises the old tracks and ties, which peek through all along the trail. Old railroad signs also line the corridor. At points, it seems little other than the actual train was removed when the line became a trail.

Pine trees provide both respite from the sun and a barrier from trailside traffic. Unfortunately, this area experiences heavy winds, and pine trees have shallow root systems, so downed trees often block the path. Those and the bumpy surface may discourage cyclists, though its flat grade accommodates walkers and joggers.

In Gilkey the Thermal Belt Rail-Trail merges with the Overmountain Victory National Historic Trail. The latter follows the route Colonial Patriots took from Virginia to join the battle at South Carolina's Kings Mountain. According to the National Park Service, 57 miles of this 330-mile trail system are open and signed. (Look for the white or brown-and-white triangular signs depicting a

Endpoints
Spindale to Gilkey

Mileage
8

Roughness Index
2

Surface
Crushed stone

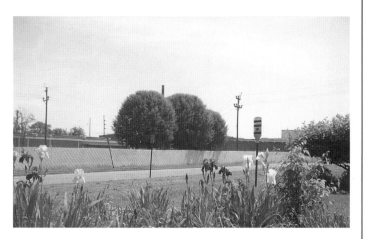

From downtown Ruth you have instant access to the Thermal Belt Rail-Trail where, further along, you can spot old tracks and ties beneath the crushed stone surface.

soldier in profile.) If you're visiting in October, you may want to check out the annual Overmountain Victory Trail March along this route.

DIRECTIONS FROM CHARLOTTE

To reach the Spindale trailhead, take I-85 South about 25 miles to Exit 10B/US Highway 74, head west about 34 miles, and turn off at ALT 74 toward Spindale. In town, turn right on Oakland Road, then left on West Main Street. The trailhead is at the intersection of West Main and Kentucky Street. Park along the road.

Contact: Rutherford County Tourism Development Authority
1990 US Highway 221 South
Forest City, NC 28043
(828) 245-1492
www.rutherfordtourism.com/links/index.php?
LID=660&LS=CList

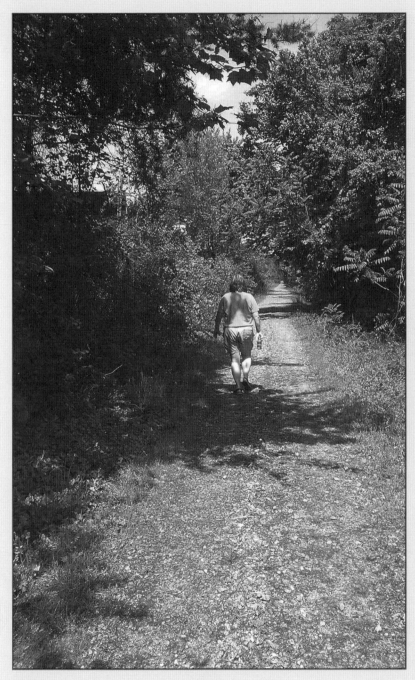

A pedestrian enjoys a wooded section of the Thermal Belt Rail-Trail near Ruth.

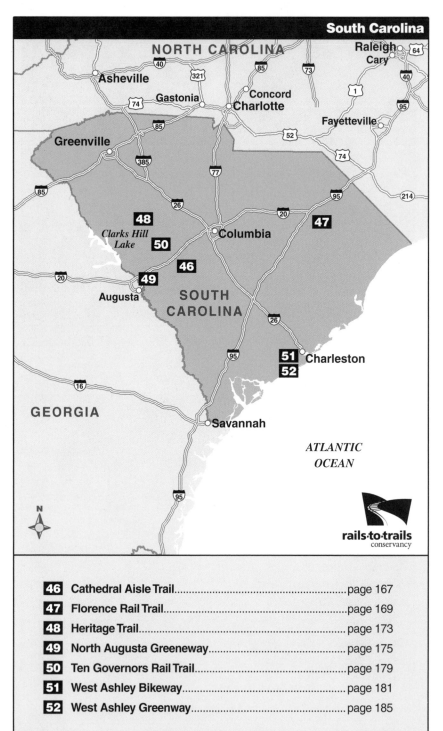

NORTH CAROLINA

Raleigh
Cary

Asheville

Gastonia

Concord
Charlotte

Fayetteville

Greenville

48

Clarks Hill
Lake

50

46

Columbia

47

49

Augusta

SOUTH
CAROLINA

51 Charleston

52

GEORGIA

Savannah

*ATLANTIC
OCEAN*

N

rails·to·trails
conservancy

South Carolina

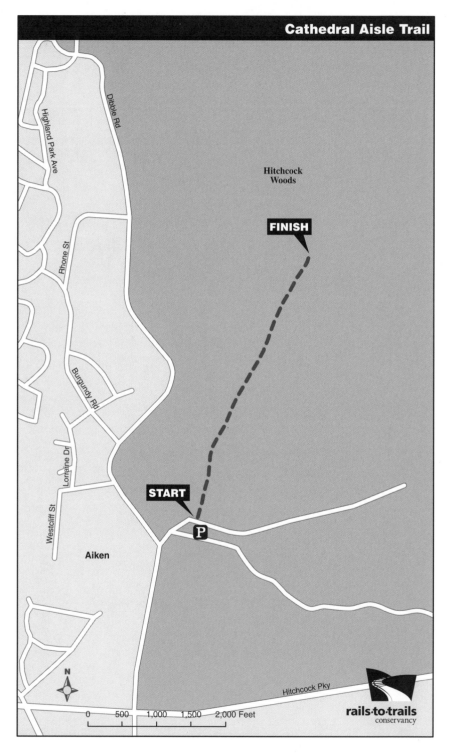

Cathedral Aisle Trail

Dibble Rd

Highland Park Ave

Hitchcock
Woods

Rhone St

FINISH

Burgundy Rd

Lorraine Dr

START

Westcliff St

P

Aiken

N

Hitchcock Pky

0   500   1,000   1,500   2,000 Feet

rails·to·trails
conservancy

Cathedral Aisle Trail

The Cathedral Aisle Trail is part of a 65-mile network within Aiken's protected Hitchcock Woods. Open since September 1939, this lush forest path is among the nation's oldest rail-trails. Though it runs just 0.8-mile, the route is a must-see for its railroading past alone.

The South Carolina Railroad & Canal Company built the corridor in 1835 as part of its Hamburg–Charleston route. At the time, the 136-mile line was the world's longest and the domain of a steam locomotive named the *Best Friend of Charleston*.

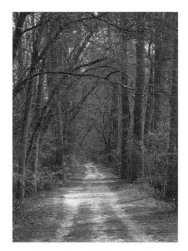

Meander through Hitchcock Woods on the Cathedral Aisle Trail, open since 1939.

In the late 1800s, Lulie and Thomas Hitchcock purchased the land surrounding the then-abandoned tracks for a hunting preserve. The Hitchcocks eventually set aside 1,200 acres for recreational purposes on condition the area never be sold to a private individual or firm. Today, through the support of donors and volunteers, the Hitchcock Foundation manages more than 2,000 acres of mature forest, ponds, streams, and wetlands. At its heart is the rail-trail.

Endpoints
Fulmer Gate/Dibble Road to Hitchcock Woods Trail

Mileage
0.8

Roughness Index
3

Surface
Dirt, sand

Cyclists are barred from the trail network, though most bikes would bog down in the soft sand anyway. You will find meandering hikers, joggers, and equestrians. You may even encounter a horse-drawn carriage on the Cathedral Aisle or connecting trails. Pick up a map at the trailhead information kiosk.

DIRECTIONS

To reach the trailhead from Aiken, take US Highway 78/Richland Avenue west to Highway 118/Hitchcock Parkway. Head south on Hitchcock about a half mile and turn left on Dibble Road. Follow Dibble just under a half mile. Parking is available in a sandy lot on the right, opposite the power station.

Contact: Aiken Chamber of Commerce
121 Richard Avenue East
Aiken, SC 29801
(803) 641-1111
www.sctrails.net/trails/alltrails/railtrails/
catheralaisle.html

Florence Rail-Trail

In 2003, the South Carolina Governor's Council on Physical Fitness recognized the Florence Rail-Trail Committee with a community award for its work on this tree-lined trail, which spans two miles between the Ebenezer Park neighborhood and nearby McLeod Health & Fitness Center. Area walkers, runners, inline skaters, and cyclists flock here for their daily fitness routines, and visitors are welcome to join them. The paved corridor provides ample room for everyone.

Replica train gates mark the trailhead at the intersection of Old Ebenezer and South Ebenezer roads. The out-and-back route passes pines, sweet gums, honeysuckle, and grape vines that host myriad birds and other critters. At trail's end, off to the right, is the fitness center, which boasts a wooded nature walk. Stroll its packed dirt trails and boardwalks that cross small streams before rejoining the rail-trail.

On National Trails Day (the first weekend of June), the fitness center hosts annual walking and running events for kids, providing registered participants with T-shirts and medals.

Endpoints
Old Ebenezer Road to McLeod Health & Fitness Center

Mileage
2

Roughness Index
1

Surface
Asphalt

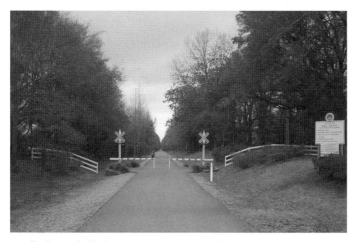

The Florence Rail-Trail is the go-to fitness destination for area walkers, runners, and cyclists.

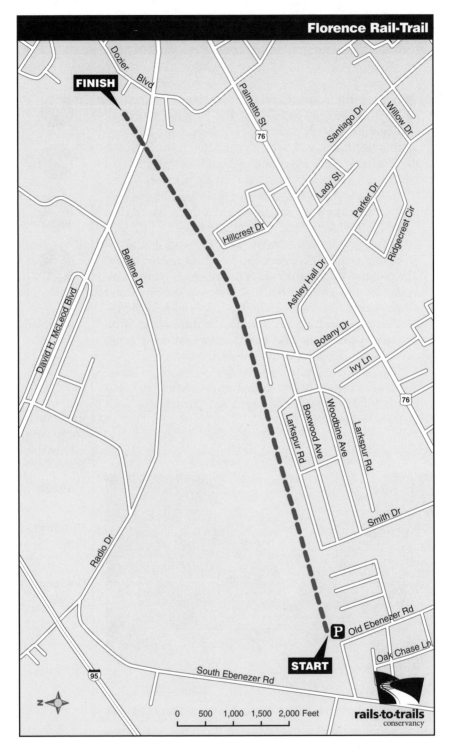

Florence Rail-Trail

FINISH

Dozier Blvd

Palmetto St

76

Santiago Dr

Willow Dr

Lady St

Parker Dr

Ridgecrest Cir

Hillcrest Dr

Beltline Dr

David H. McLeod Blvd

Ashley Hall Dr

Botany Dr

Ivy Ln

76

Larkspur Rd

Boxwood Ave

Woodbine Ave

Larkspur Rd

Radio Dr

Smith Dr

Old Ebenezer Rd

P

Oak Chase Ln

START

South Ebenezer Rd

95

N

0   500   1,000   1,500   2,000 Feet

rails·to·trails
conservancy

DIRECTIONS

Take I-95 to Exit 157 and head east on US Highway 76. After about a mile, turn left on South Ebenezer Road, then right on Old Ebenezer Road, just shy of the trailhead. Parking is on the left.

Contact: City of Florence Recreation Department
P.O. Box 1476
Florence, SC 29503
(843) 665-3253
www.sctrails.net/trails/alltrails/railtrails/
florencerail.html

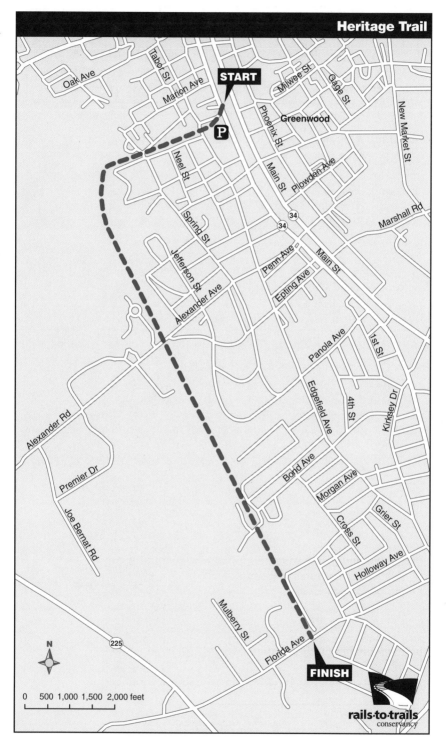

START

P

Greenwood

FINISH

0 500 1,000 1,500 2,000 feet

N

rails·to·trails
conservancy

Heritage Trail

There's no better place to take in Greenwood's industrial and railroading past than along the aptly named Heritage Trail, which extends more than two miles from the town center south to outlying countryside. Through the mid-20th century five railroads ran through town, crisscrossing and paralleling each other. (This route runs along the Georgia & Florida Railroad corridor.) The busy junction was dubbed Hobo Jungle, as the rails attracted a population of transients who would captivate local children with tales of wayward adventure.

A commemorative brick plaza marks the trailhead. It centers on a turntable once used by railroad workers, two at a time, to manually turn steam locomotives for their return trips. The plaza also holds interpretive signs, a pair of passenger cars from the early 1900s, and the Railroad Historical Center.

A half mile along the tree-lined trail, look for the old Coca-Cola building, which bottled pop through the 1950s. In the early 20th century a circus set up its tents in the adjacent field, and the rail line was used to transport animals and equipment for a downtown parade. Farther

Endpoints
Main Street to
Florida Avenue,
Greenwood

Mileage
2.5

Roughness Index
1

Surface
Asphalt

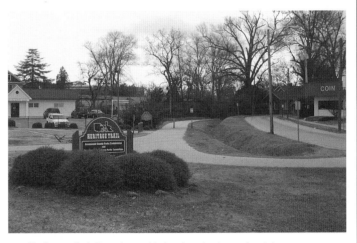

The Heritage Trail offers a historical look at the railroad it was founded on.

173

down the trail stand the century-old Panola and Mathews mills, part of the nationwide Abney Mills and Greenwood Mills textile companies. On the west side of the trail, the Grede Foundry still casts automobile parts and other products. The paved trail ends amid open fields and scattered homes.

DIRECTIONS

Take I-26 to Exit 54 and head southwest on SC 72 about 30 miles to Cambridge Avenue in Greenwood. Veer right on US Highway 25 Business to Main Street/SC 34. The trailhead is at the intersection of Main and Circular Avenue. Palmetto Bank allows trail users to park in its lot.

Contact: Greater Greenwood Parks & Trails Foundation
P.O. Box 8021
Greenwood, SC 29649
(864) 229-8018
www.sctrails.net/trails/alltrails/railtrails/heritage.html

North Augusta Greeneway

Referred to locally as the Greeneway, this trail meanders more than five miles through the riverfront community of North Augusta, from The River Golf Club on the Savannah River through residential neighborhoods and wooded alcoves to its western terminus at Pisgah Road. Despite the dense suburban setting, a careful trail design engenders a surprisingly natural environment.

Buffering much of the route is a 100-foot-wide, wooded right-of-way that provides habitat for native birds. Trees hide more developed sections of the trail, while tunnels whisk users beneath busy road crossings. Such conscientious environmental planning has earned the Greeneway federal designation as a National Recreation Trail.

Residents use the Greeneway as a travel corridor between surrounding neighborhoods. If you're just visiting, the trail offers a great way to explore the area. Hop on and mingle with locals out for a ride or a stroll. Roll into Hammond Hill skate park, south of the trail on Cypress Drive in Riverview Park, and watch as skateboarders hone their skills. If you're interested in more relaxing pursuits, head to the fishing pier on the Savannah, a short walk from the Riverview trailhead.

Endpoints
River Club Golf Course to Pisgah Road

Mileage
5.3

Roughness Index
1

Surface
Asphalt

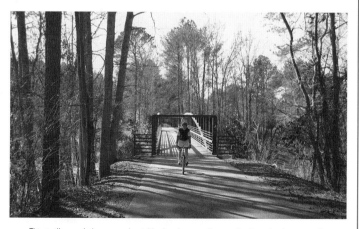

This trail's wooded areas and neighborhood connections make it a valued community asset.

175

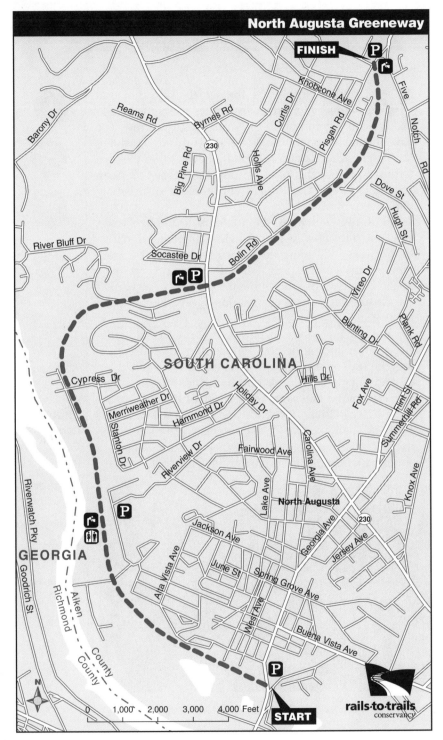

North Augusta Greeneway

FINISH

Knobcone Ave

Five Notch Rd

Curtis Dr

Reams Rd

Byrnes Rd

Pisgah Rd

Barony Dr

Big Pine Rd

230

Hollis Ave

Dove St

Hugh St

River Bluff Dr

Socastee Dr

Bolin Rd

Vireo Dr

Plank Rd

Bunting Dr

SOUTH CAROLINA

Hills Dr

Cypress Dr

Fox Ave

Flint St

Merriweather Dr

Hammond Dr

Holiday Dr

Summerhill Rd

Stanton Dr

Riverview Dr

Fairwood Ave

Carolina Ave

Knox Ave

Riverwatch Pky

North Augusta

Lake Ave

Georgia Ave

230

Jackson Ave

Jersey Ave

GEORGIA

Goodrich St

Ala Vista Ave

June St

Spring Grove Ave

Buena Vista Ave

West Ave

Aiken County

Richmond County

N

0   1,000   2,000   3,000   4,000 Feet

START

rails·to·trails
conservancy

DIRECTIONS

To reach the Riverview Park trailhead from Georgia Avenue in North Augusta, take Buena Vista Avenue west, turn left on Georgetown Drive, and continue to the activities center parking lot in Riverview Park. This access point links up with the trail just over a mile north of The River Golf Club trailhead.

Contact: North Augusta Parks, Recreation & Leisure Services
P.O. Box 6400
North Augusta, SC 29861
(803) 441-4300
www.northaugusta.net/Dept_Serv/Parks_Recre/
greeneway.html

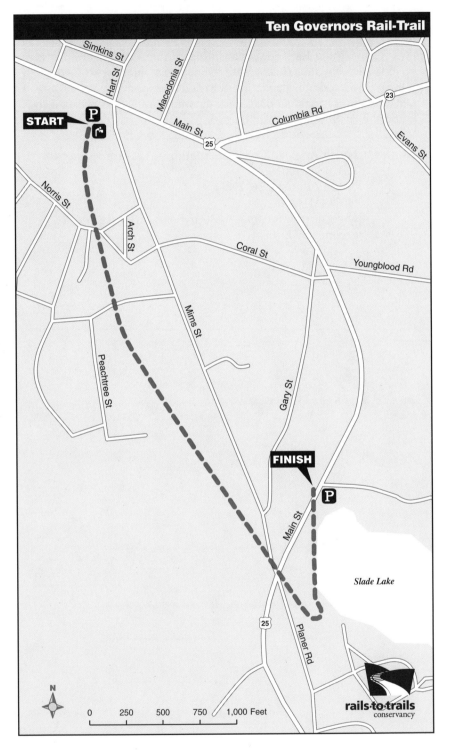

Ten Governors Rail-Trail

Ten Governors Rail-Trail

The town of Edgefield has taken pride in the political initiative of its native sons for nearly 200 years and today dubs itself the "Home of Ten Governors." This legacy began in 1816 with Gov. Andrew Pickens, II, who was instrumental in the construction of South Carolina's roads and canals. Perhaps the best known of those hailing from Edgefield was James Strom Thurmond (1902–2003), a state governor, presidential candidate, and oldest person ever to serve in the U.S. senate. Thurmond retired in 2003 at age 100 and passed away in Edgefield six months later.

To learn more about Thurmond and his hometown gubernatorial predecessors, your best bet is to hit the Ten Governors Rail-Trail. Stretching from town nearly a mile southeast to Slade Lake, the trail features 10 granite markers, each providing a biographical narrative of a governor hailing from the area. Like many rail-trails, this one is popular with walkers, runners, inline skaters, and cyclists. What sets it apart, aside from history, is that it remains lighted and open for 24-hour use.

Endpoints
Main Street to
Slade Lake,
Edgefield

Mileage
0.9

**Roughness
Index**
1

Surface
Asphalt

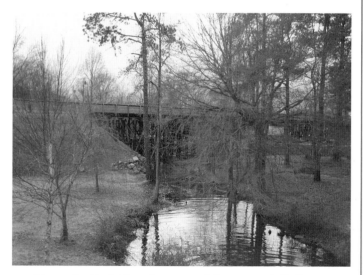

A former railroad trestle takes trail users over a small waterway on the Ten Governors Rail-Trail.

179

From the trailhead parking area at Main and Mims streets, the 10-foot-wide paved path winds past ballparks, neighborhoods, and trailside benches before crossing a long wooden bridge (formerly a railroad trestle). The otherwise flat trail descends steeply for a short stretch, then curves toward Slade Lake, where it skirts the shore along a bridge. The lake's fishing pier and boat launch are open to the public (fishing permitted on Wednesdays and weekends between April and November).

DIRECTIONS

Take I-20 to Exit 18 and head north on SC 19/Edgefield Highway. In Trenton, SC 19 becomes US Highway 25/Augusta Road, which enters downtown Edgefield as Main Street. Park in the lot on the south side of the Main and Mims Street intersection.

Contact: Town of Edgefield
400 Main Street
Edgefield, SC 29824
(803) 637-4014
www.sctrails.net/trails/alltrails/railtrails/
tengovernors.html

West Ashley Bikeway

Running arrow-straight from the Ashley River west to a wholesale produce stand on Wappoo Road, the West Ashley Bikeway links several suburban Charleston neighborhoods, providing a 2.5-mile cycling and walking path.

Initial plans called for an entirely different corridor. After the Seaboard Coastline Railroad abandoned the line in 1976, the state wanted to build an expressway along the route. When that plan fell through, the City of Charleston negotiated to lease the corridor from the state for $1 a year and completed the trail in 1983.

While the route rolls along largely unobstructed, it is sparsely maintained and marred by one particularly hazardous intersection. Leaving the riverfront, pedestrians must negotiate busy, four-lane St. Andrews Boulevard without benefit of a light or crosswalk. Use extreme caution when crossing.

Endpoints
Ashley River to
Wappoo Road

Mileage
2.5

Roughness Index
1

Surface
Asphalt

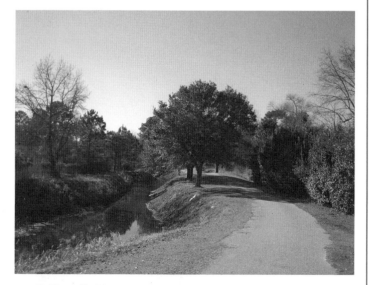

The West Ashley Bikeway runs along the raised berm of the former Seaboard Coastline Railroad.

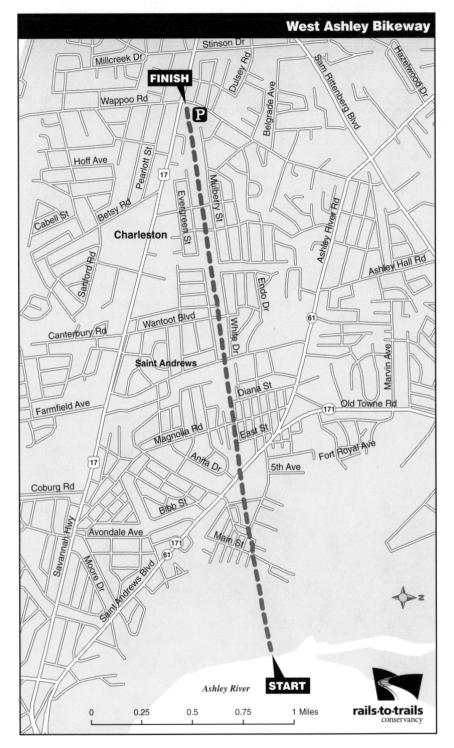

West Ashley Bikeway

FINISH

P

Stinson Dr

Millcreek Dr

Dulsey Rd

Sam Rittenberg Blvd

Hazelwood Dr

Wappoo Rd

Belgrade Ave

Hoff Ave

Pearlott St

17

Mulberry St

Betsy Rd

Evergreen St

Cabell St

Sanford Rd

Charleston

Ashley River Rd

Ashley Hall Rd

Endo Dr

Wantoot Blvd

Canterbury Rd

White Dr

61

Saint Andrews

Marvin Ave

Farmfield Ave

Diana St

171

Old Towne Rd

Magnolia Rd

East St

Anita Dr

Fort Royal Ave

17

5th Ave

Coburg Rd

Bibb St

Savannah Hwy

Moore Dr

Avondale Ave

171

61

Saint Andrews Blvd

Main St

N

Ashley River

START

0   0.25   0.5   0.75   1 Miles

rails·to·trails
conservancy

DIRECTIONS

To reach the Wappoo Road trailhead from downtown Charleston, take US Highway 17 west across the Ashley River Memorial Bridge, continue three miles, and turn right on Wappoo Road. Within 50 yards, look for a small produce stand on the right, adjacent to the trailhead. Park in the gravel lot.

To reach the Ashley River trailhead, just past the bridge turn right on SC 61/SC 171/St. Andrews Boulevard and look for a trailhead sign just before SC 61 and SC 171 split.

Contact: Charleston Department of Parks
30 Mary Murray Drive
Charleston, SC 29403
(843) 724-7321
www.sctrails.net/trails/alltrails/railtrails/
westashbikeway.html

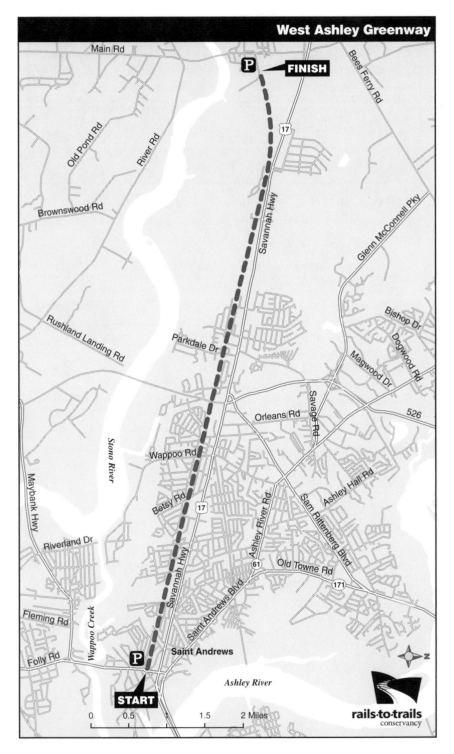

West Ashley Greenway

West Ashley Greenway

A favorite of local mountain bikers, the West Ashley Greenway takes you on a 10.5-mile out-and-back ride from suburban Charleston west to the scenic Lowcountry wetlands that surround this charming city.

From its trailhead behind the South Windermere Shopping Center, the greenway connects several miles of subdivisions on a 100-foot-wide packed-dirt path. On Johns Island, the dirt gives way to rough gravel and narrow bridge crossings—mountain bikes are a must for this section. Here the broad wetlands flank the trail, presenting magnificent views and rewarding bird sightings. If your timing is right, you may catch sight of the tidal flow that carved these lacework channels.

The agricultural heart of the region, Johns Island is the nation's largest producer of tomatoes. In fact, much of the fresh produce served in local restaurants hails from this still rural but slowly developing community. (Don't tell the folks in South Georgia, but the island's Wadmalaw sweet onions are said to rival Vidalias in flavor.)

Endpoints
South Windemere
Shopping Center
to Johns Island,
Charleston

Mileage
10.5

Roughness Index
2

Surface
Dirt, gravel

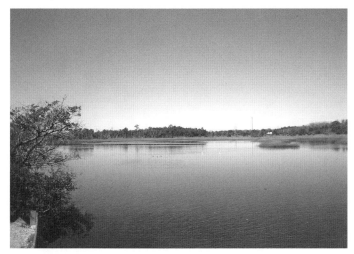

The broad Stono River flows near the West Ashley Greenway, most of which is adjacent to US Highway 17.

DIRECTIONS

To reach the trailhead from downtown Charleston, take US Highway 17 west across the Ashley River Memorial Bridge. A half mile past the bridge turn left on Folly Road. At the second light, turn right on Windermere Boulevard and enter the South Windermere Shopping Center. Park beside the trailhead on the north side of the shopping center.

Contact: Charleston Department of Parks
30 Mary Murray Drive
Charleston, SC 29403
(843) 724-7321
www.sctrails.net/trails/alltrails/railtrails/
westashgreenway.html

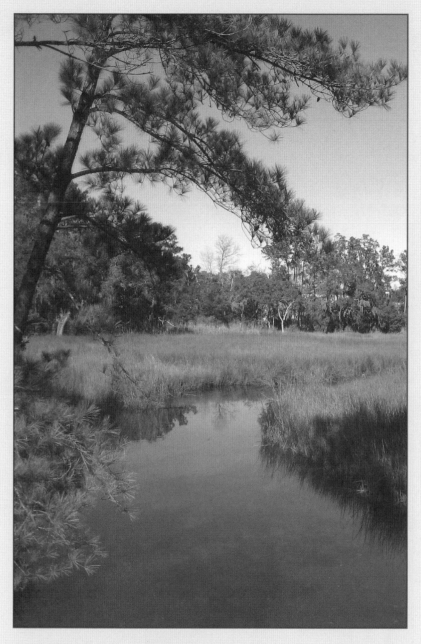

Evergreens and wetlands characterize the West Ashley Greenway.

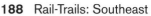

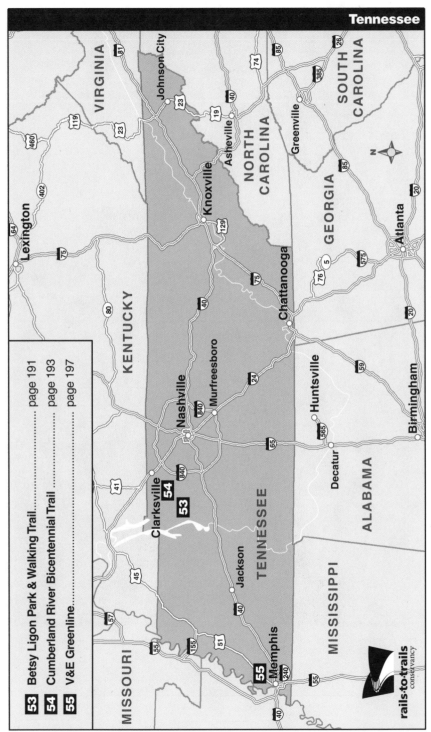

Tennessee

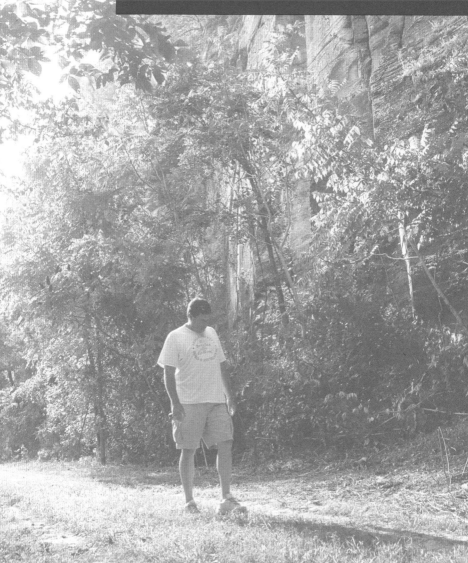

Tennessee

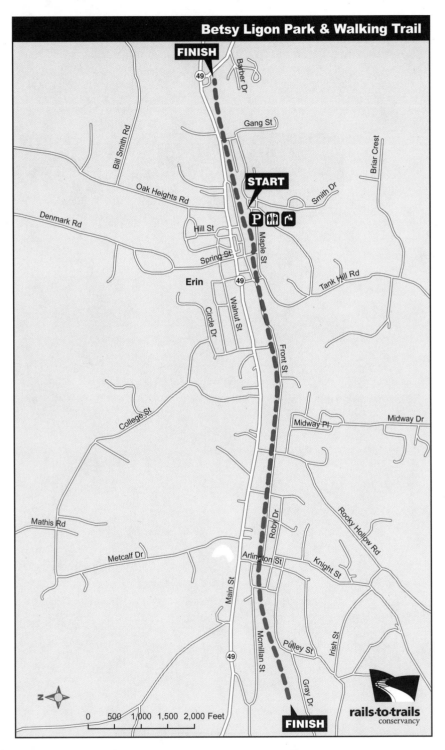

Betsy Ligon Park & Walking Trail

FINISH

49

Barber Dr

Gang St

Bill Smith Rd

Briar Crest

Oak Heights Rd

START

P

Smith Dr

Denmark Rd

Hill St

Maple St

Spring St

Erin

49

Tank Hill Rd

Circle Dr

Walnut St

Front St

College St

Midway Pl

Midway Dr

Mathis Rd

Roby Dr

Rocky Hollow Rd

Metcalf Dr

Arlington St

Knight St

Main St

Mcmillan St

Pulley St

Irish St

Gray Dr

49

N

0 500 1,000 1,500 2,000 Feet

FINISH

rails·to·trails
conservancy

Betsy Ligon Park & Walking Trail

The Betsy Ligon Park & Walking Trail is the toast of small-town Erin—just ask its namesake. At the trail opening in 1995, then Mayor Betsy Ligon was hopeful the path would provide citizens with ample space to exercise and visit with neighbors while also celebrating the town's railroading past. Her wish has been realized.

Founded by Irish railroad workers, Erin celebrates its heritage the third Saturday in March with a parade that ends in Betsy Ligon Park. Here you'll find a restored boxcar and caboose, the Railroad Memorial Pavilion, and a hand-hewn limestone kiln built in the late 1800s. Leading away from the park in either direction, the trail has become especially popular with the senior set, who take advantage of its smooth paved surface and safe surroundings to keep fit.

Beyond the town center, trees and birds replace people and cars as the backdrop to your ride or stroll. Several benches along the way beckon you to slow down, relax, and contemplate the natural surroundings. Plans call for extending the trail beyond the city limits, and from the looks of the well-worn footpath along the undeveloped corridor, the trailblazing has begun.

Endpoints
Within Erin

Mileage
2

Roughness Index
1

Surface
Asphalt

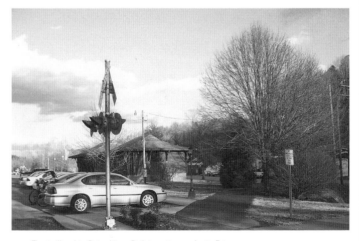

The trailhead in Betsy Ligon Park is quite popular in Erin.

DIRECTIONS

Erin lies some 50 miles west of Nashville. As you enter town along Main Street/Highway 49, turn south on Hill Street and follow it 0.2 mile to Front Street. Park at the Front Street entrance to the Railroad Memorial Pavilion in Betsy Ligon Park.

Contact: Erin City Hall
P.O. Box 270
Erin, TN 37061
(931) 289-4108
www.tnvacation.com/vendors/
betsy_ligon_park_and_walking_trail

Cumberland River Bicentennial Trail

Whether you're after a picnic, a leisurely stroll, or a brisk bike ride, the 6.5-mile Cumberland River Bicentennial Trail (a.k.a. Ashland City Rail-Trail) will enchant you as it meanders past lively streams and waterfalls, across misty wetlands, and atop jagged bluffs along the Cumberland River. Only 20 minutes northwest of downtown Nashville, it connects users with the great outdoors along two adjoining segments.

A mile north of town, the Marks Creek trailhead offers parking, portable toilets, and helpful trail signage. Here begins the Trestle Bridge trail section, an Ashland City park since 1997. This paved, wheelchair-accessible corridor runs four miles northwest to the Sycamore Harbor trailhead. The first mile leads past trickling waterfalls and spring dogwood blooms to the Turkey Junction Native Gardens & Comfort Station, a great spot to relax and refuel.

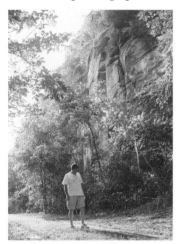

On the more remote section of the Cumberland River Bicentennial Trail, limestone bluffs and a breeze off the river keep the trail cool.

The route threads past secluded lakes and a designated waterfowl area to an impressive railroad bridge. One of six original trestles along the trail, it offers sweeping views of the wetlands that border the Cumberland River. The trail soon ends at the Sycamore Harbor trailhead on Chapmansboro Road.

From its trailhead on Chapmansboro Road, the Eagle Pass trail section runs 2.5 miles through equally beautiful surroundings to the Cheatham Lock and Dam campground. Its compacted gravel surface is unsuitable for road bikes, so strap on your hiking boots or hop on your mountain bike. To extend your trek, pitch a tent at the campground and save the return trip for another day.

Endpoints
Marks Creek, Sycamore Harbor & Cheatham Lock and Dam campground, Ashland City

Mileage
6.5

Roughness Index
1

Surface
Asphalt

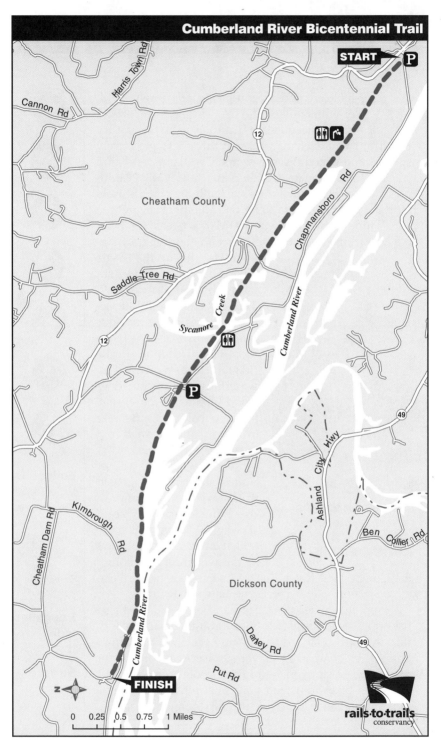

Cumberland River Bicentennial Trail

START

Harris Town Rd

Cannon Rd

12

Chapmansboro Rd

Cheatham County

Saddle Tree Rd

Sycamore Creek

Cumberland River

12

49

Cheatham Dam Rd

Kimbrough Rd

Ashland City Hwy

Ben Collier Rd

Dickson County

Darley Rd

49

Cumberland River

Put Rd

N

FINISH

0   0.25   0.5   0.75   1 Miles

rails·to·trails
conservancy

DIRECTIONS FROM NASHVILLE

Take I-40 West to Exit 204 and head north on Highway 155/Briley Parkway. At Exit 24 take Highway 12/Hydes Ferry Pike/Ashland City Highway about 13 miles west into town.

Or take I-24 West to Exit 24 and head south on Highway 49 about 10 miles to Ashland City.

To reach the Marks Creek trailhead, take Highway 12 about a mile north of town. Just past the bridge by the Deerfield Inn, turn left on Chapmansboro Road. The marked trailhead is on the right.

Contact: Ashland City Parks & Recreation Department
233 Tennessee Waltz Parkway, Suite 101
Ashland City, TN 37015
(615) 792-2655
www.cheathamchamber.org/trail

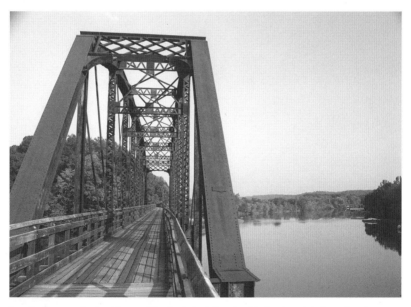

Spanning Sycamore Creek, a tributary of the Cumberland River, the old railroad trestle is the perfect place to spot waterfowl, river otters, and beavers.

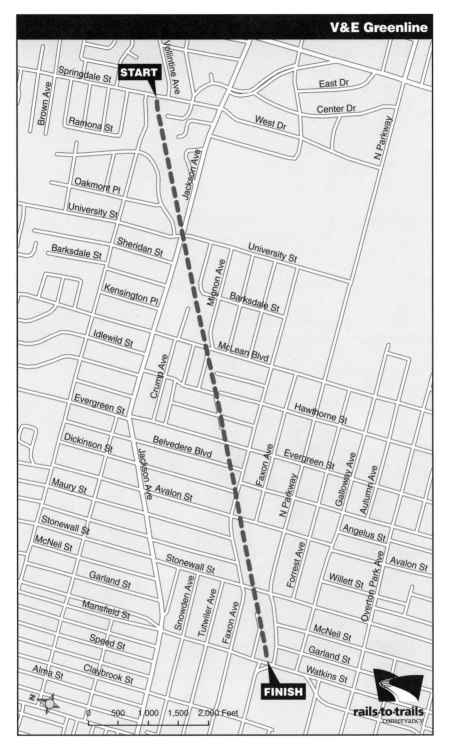

V&E Greenline

START

Springdale St

Brown Ave

Vollintine Ave

East Dr

Center Dr

West Dr

N Parkway

Ramona St

Jackson Ave

Oakmont Pl

University St

Sheridan St

University St

Barksdale St

Mignon Ave

Kensington Pl

Barksdale St

Idlewild St

McLean Blvd

Crump Ave

Evergreen St

Hawthorne St

Dickinson St

Belvedere Blvd

Faxon Ave

Evergreen St

Galloway Ave

Autumn Ave

Jackson Ave

Maury St

Avalon St

N Parkway

Stonewall St

McNeil St

Angelus St

Stonewall St

Forrest Ave

Willett St

Overton Park Ave

Avalon St

Garland St

Snowden Ave

Tutwiler Ave

Faxon Ave

Mansfield St

McNeil St

Speed St

Garland St

Alma St

Claybrook St

Watkins St

FINISH

N

0   500   1,000   1,500   2,000 Feet

rails·to·trails
conservancy

V&E Greenline

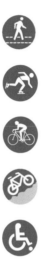

It has been said that it "takes a village" to build a rail-trail. In the case of the 1.7-mile V&E Greenline, the village in question is the Vollintine-Evergreen neighborhood. Banding together in the mid-1990s to transform the abandoned railroad corridor into a public green space, this Memphis community continues to maintain and improve the popular trail. During regular Spruce up the Greenline days, volunteers remove debris, rake leaves, plant trees, and tend community gardens along this verdant route.

A perfect outlet for those seeking a quiet retreat from city life, the trail provides a safe haven for walkers, runners, and cyclists. The route comprises eight contiguous sections: the Springs, the Cut, the Gardens, the Arbors, Lick Creek, Utility Park, West Creek, and the West End.

From the east, the shady Springs segment runs between Springdale Street and Jackson Avenue, emerging from the tree canopy on the Cut, a sunken segment where native plants and invasive kudzu do battle. Across McLean is the Gardens, where more than 30

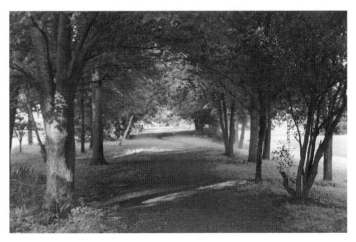

The V&E Greenline's multiple gardens lend it a southern plantation feel.

Endpoints
Springdale Street
to Watkins Street
and North Parkway,
Memphis

Mileage
1.7

Roughness Index
2

Surface
Ballast, Grass, Dirt

197

flower varieties showcase their vibrant colors between February and November. Stop and smell the flowers before continuing to the Arbors, which boasts 15 tree species. Volunteers transplanted many of the latter in July 2003 after hurricane-force winds destroyed hundreds of area trees.

Next in line, Lick Creek, Utility Park, and West Creek center on human-made highlights. Adjacent to Auburndale and Evergreen streets, Lick Creek Bridge was built with local help by Keeler Iron Works to replace the original span, which was removed when the railroad stopped running. Utility Park is an oak-dotted flat that borders a Memphis Light, Gas & Water pumping facility. West Creek Bridge runs behind the Woodmont Towers apartment complex, providing residents with easy trail access.

The route ends at Watkins Street and North Parkway in West End, where residential homes line flanking slopes. Take a stroll along this leafy oasis, and you'll understand the parental pride of its urban keepers.

DIRECTIONS

To reach the trailhead at Watkins Street and North Parkway, take the I-40/I-240 Expressway to the North Parkway exit and head west four blocks to its intersection with Watkins. Street parking is available.

To reach the trail's eastern end at Springdale Street, follow the above directions, turn left on Watkins, and drive four blocks to Jackson Avenue. Turn right on Jackson, drive about 1.5 miles, and turn left on Springdale. The trail access point is one block up. Street parking is available.

Contact: Vollintine-Evergreen Community
1680 Jackson Avenue
Memphis, TN 38107
(901) 276-1782
www.vegreenline.org

STAFF PICKS

Best Rail-Trails

When Rails-to-Trails Conservancy staff members scoured the Southeast for great rail-trails, these were the ones that stood out as the best. Short or long, city or country, these are rail-trails not to miss.

Alabama

Chief Ladiga Trail

Florida

Fred Marquis Pinellas Trail

Jacksonville–Baldwin Rail-Trail

Seminole Wekiva Trail

Tallahassee–St. Marks Historic
    Railroad State Trail

West Orange Trail

Withlacoochee State Trail

Georgia

Augusta Canal Trail

Silver Comet Trail

Mississippi

Longleaf Trace

North Carolina

Charlotte Trolley Rail-with-Trail

Greensboro Rail-Trail System

South Carolina

North Augusta Greeneway

Tennessee

Cumberland River
    Bicentennial Trail

For History Buffs

These rail-trails don't just challenge your body, they challenge your mind. Pick up some historical tidbits on these trails.

Alabama

Chattahoochee Valley
    Railroad Trail

Richard Martin Trail

Georgia

Augusta Canal Trail

McQueens Island Historic Trail

North Carolina

Gold Hill Rail-Trail

South Carolina

Cathedral Aisle Trail

Ten Governors Rail-Trail

Tennessee

Cumberland River
    Bicentennial Trail

ACKNOWLEDGMENTS

Each of the trails in *Rail-Trails: Southeast* was personally visited by Rails-to-Trails Conservancy staff. Maps, photographs, and trail descriptions are as accurate as possible thanks to the work of the following contributors:

Barbara Richey
Ben Carter
Billy Fields
Franz Gimmler
Frederick Schaedtler
Gene Olig
Heather Deutsch
Jeff Ciabotti
Jessica Leas
Jessica Tump
Kelly Cornell
Ken Bryan
Marianne Fowler
Meghan Taylor

Special thanks to all the trail managers we called upon for assistance in preparing this guidebook. Our sincere thanks to Terry Peek, director of Moultrie-Colquitt County Parks & Recreation Department for collecting GIS data of the Moultrie Trail in Georgia.

 Special thanks to Coca-Cola North America and American Express Company for their generous support that helped make this guidebook possible.

INDEX

Note: Page numbers in **boldface** indicate main rail-trail listings.

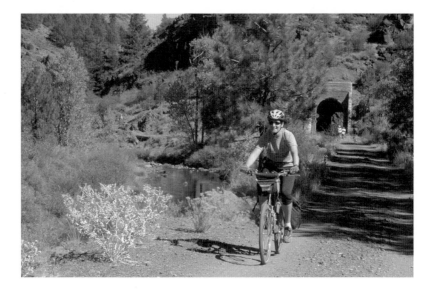

Become a member
of Rails-to-Trails Conservancy

As the nation's leader in helping communities transform unused railroad corridor into multi-use trails, Rails-to-Trails Conservancy (RTC) depends on the support of its members and donors to create access to healthy outdoor experiences.

You can help secure the future of rail-trails and enhance America's communities and countryside by becoming a member of Rails-to-Trails Conservancy today. Your donations will help support programs, projects and services that have helped put more than 13,000 rail-trail miles on the ground.

Every day, RTC provides vital technical assistance to communities throughout the country, advocates for trail-friendly policies at the local, state and national level, promotes the benefits of rail-trails and defends rail-trail laws in the courts.

Join RTC in *"inspiring movement"* and receive the following benefits:

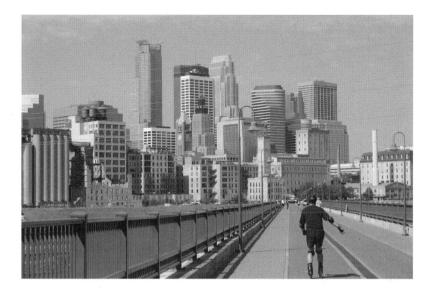

❶ New member welcome materials including *Destination Rail-Trails*, a sampler of some of the nation's finest trails

❷ A **subscription** to RTC's quarterly magazine, *Rails to Trails.*

❸ **Discounts** on publications, apparel and other merchandise including RTC's popular rail-trail guidebooks.

❹ The **satisfaction** of knowing that your dollars are helping to create a nationwide network of trails.

Membership benefits start at just $18, but additional contributions are gladly accepted.

Join online at **www.railstotrails.org**

Join by mail by sending your contribution to Rails-to-Trails Conservancy, Attention: Membership, 1100 17th St. NW, 10th Floor, Washington, DC 20036.

Join by phone by calling 1-866-202-9788.

Contributions to Rails-to-Trails Conservancy are tax deductible to the full extent of the law.